THE LITMUS PAPERS

A National Health Dis-Service

First published November 1980
by Centre for Policy Studies
8 Wilfred Street, London S.W.1

Typeset and printed by
Orchard & Ind Ltd.
104 Northgate Street, Gloucester

ISBN 0-905880-28-5

Contents

(Continued)

Introduction and Acknowledgements

Introduction and Acknowledgements

For the radical reforms that are long overdue in the NHS to be expected and welcomed by the public, better understanding of its defects is a first essential.

For many years it has been difficult to write candidly about the NHS because of the emotions generated in favour of a "Service" designed to serve the public without regard to cost, income or wealth. But it has had over 30 years to produce the results claimed for it by Aneurin Bevan and its Founding Fathers in all three political parties. For some years individual doctors have left the NHS to practise overseas or in Britain privately. Individual observers – economists and others – have pointed to failures and defects. In more recent times the public itself has protested against long queues or years of waiting, against harassed doctors with too little time to listen to symptoms or explain treatment, against the neglect or maltreatment of the old and mentally sick in hospital. But there is still no strong public demand for reform.

The advent of a government prepared to consider radical solutions provides the timing of this collection of essays. Its object is to inform and arouse public opinion to the urgency of reform. It deals mainly with the long-suppressed defects of the NHS. The solutions remain to be worked out and tried out, initially perhaps on a small scale to see how they work. In this way they will avoid the tragic mistake of the NHS, itself a vast structure, imposed on the whole country, that soon generated vested interests which obstruct reform however bad its results.

A better public understanding is a pre-requisite for long-overdue change. Government can lead, but the obstructions to reform – from the central bureaucracy to local interests – make it essential to create an informed public opinion that will want government to over-ride the obstructors.

This collection does not claim to be a comprehensive dissection of the NHS; the gaps will perhaps be filled by others later. Still less does it attempt a blueprint for alternative health systems, though some essays indicate general principles along which reform could proceed. What it does show, in moods varying from dispassionate analysis to disappointed anger, sadness and frustration, that the standards of efficiency and service in an institution in which hopes had been raised so high by its founders should have sunk so low.

We are indebted to the writers of these essays – three family doctors, eight specialists, nine economists, two sociologists, two insurance experts: twenty men, four women – for contributing their expertise. Each has written in a personal capacity, independent of any organisation or firm, and without commitment to the political outlook of the Centre for Policy Study.

In particular, we are most grateful to George Bunton, Chairman of the Centre's Health Study Group, and to Arthur Seldon, for the time they have so willingly and voluntarily given to inspiring, guiding and co-ordinating these essays.

Hugh Thomas
Chairman
Centre for Policy Studies

I
The NHS
Success? Still on Trial? Failure?

Arthur Seldon

Co-director of the Institute of Economic Affairs since its early years. First Class Honours graduate of the London School of Economics; has been tutor in economics to the University of London and staff examiner in economics. Has specialised in the economics of the welfare state and of market-based welfare services. Special Adviser to a Cabinet Committee on Welfare of the Commonwealth Government of Australia, 1968. Sat on the BMA Advisory Committee on Health Services Financing, 1968–70. Numerous writings on health economics.

"The envy of the world"
"The NHS is, and will remain for many years, a complicated experiment . . ."
"There was never a case for a permanent, all-embracing NHS."

These are the three broad views about the NHS between which the British people can choose. I emphasise the choice is for the British people to make. They are a sovereign people. The formation of the NHS in 1948 was a political act of government. It was said to have the support of people in all three main political parties. But if public opinion were now convinced that the NHS had failed, or that it had had a long enough trial and should not be allowed to stop trials of other health systems, no politicians would be justified in preventing their opinion from being given effect.

1. The envy of the world?

The first view is that of Mrs Barbara Castle and others who think the NHS principle of providing medical care free at the time it is supplied is the ultimate in wisdom. Whatever its failings or drawbacks they envisage the NHS as a new system that began in 1948 and is here to stay for ever. They believe the defects can be removed by reconstruction, or more tax money, or total exclusion of private medicine. In any event, never again are people to be expected to pay for medicine when they are ill, but only through taxes on their pay and purchases when not ill.

There are three obvious errors (among many) in this reasoning.

First, paying by taxing is not the only way of paying when you are not ill. The same can be done by annual premiums for ordinary private insurance. On the other hand, paying nothing when you are ill (whether in the NHS or to a private doctor) is not an undiluted blessing. It may be the best method for emergencies; even then when you have recovered you are normally capable of knowing what you are paying for. But in non-emergency medical services – the large majority – paying is a good way of telling you what they cost and discouraging thoughtless use of busy doctors and nurses required for urgent illness.

Secondly, the NHS is, of course, not free. But making it *appear* free destroys the patient's bargaining power with the doctor. If he pays, directly or indirectly through insurance, he can usually take his custom elsewhere.

Thirdly, it is foolish to suppose there can never be anything better than the NHS. We simply do not know when somebody may think of a better way of paying for medical care. So there is never a case for a monopoly NHS to last for ever and to have the power to exclude all other methods of paying.

Of Western countries only Italy has "copied" the NHS. Its scheme began on 1 January 1980 – on paper. And there is early talk of early reform. [Essay XXI]

2. A very long experiment?

The second view is quoted from Lord Taylor who, as Dr Stephen Taylor, helped Aneurin Bevan inaugurate the NHS.

This, at least, is a more sensible view than the first: it recognises that the NHS is only an "experiment", that it is still on trial, and that it has not yet proved itself superior to all other methods.

But it is still unjustifiably optimistic that the NHS will one day prove itself. How do we know? Lord Taylor says 'for many more years?' How many is that? The NHS has already had 32. Is it to have 10 more or 20 more or 30?

When shall we be able to say, 'enough is enough'? The NHS has had a long trial. It still suffers from faults (for example, large regional differences) it was supposed to have abolished in its early years. And it has developed new faults no one dreamed of in 1948 (queueing, waiting months or years for treatment, maltreatment of the old and mentally ill in hospital, harassed and overworked doctors, British-trained doctors lost by emigration, etc.). How much longer are we to wait for the idyllic result – the best medicine for everyone, in Bevin's euphoria – to appear? Are we never to supplement or supplant it with other systems that might work better? – or at least try other systems?

Lord Taylor is uneasy that all may not have gone well. He is very severe on people who would make the NHS a tightly-closed, exclusive institution. He now wants all kinds of things that people like Mrs Castle would denounce – not least, that doctors be able to treat private patients in NHS hospitals. He wants the ultimate blasphemy – he envisages, 'as a challenge [to the NHS] rather than a disaster . . . the creation of an independent health service alongside the National Health Service . . .' to break the state monopoly. And he offers the example of ITV competition to the BBC which, he says, has improved both.

Whatever Lord Taylor may now say, this world *of comparison by competition* was certainly not envisaged by those around Bevan in 1948. The notion then was that the NHS would prove to be so good that no one in Britain would ever want anything else. Now Lord Taylor, one of the Founding Fathers, says *it must have the stimulus of competition from* private *medicine*.

Lord Taylor says he still believes in the NHS and that it can be saved if decentralised to regional control. But that declaration of faith now hardly rings true. For if the "independent" health service proves better than the NHS, will it be suppressed? If people prefer it to the NHS, will they be stopped from transferring their money to it?

He may be right: regional control *might* save the NHS from centralised seizure. He cannot know he is right. He can only speculate. But he can hardly expect the whole of the NHS to be reconstructed on regional lines in the *hope* that he is right.

For how many years would the regional theory have to be tried to judge whether it can save the NHS? Ten years? Twenty? Another thirty? And does the whole populace have to endure the same system with all its familiar faults?

The most he can expect is a *small* trial for a *short* period, say for three years in North Wales where he lives. Even that would be expensive if, as I expect, it failed because it simply decentralises *political* control instead of replacing it with *patient*-power based on personal payment.

And if Lord Taylor claimed that a small, short trial would be inadequate, he might again be right. No one would know. But he would be doing better than other people with ideas – like some in these essays – that are not being tried at all.

Yet even Lord Taylor's regional solution, it seems, will not be tried in the NHS. It was turned down by the 1979 Merrison Royal Commission. And Lord Taylor thinks the reason was that the DHSS officials considered the NHS had become too centralised and there was no going back on all that.

Lord Taylor cannot really complain that his main idea – the NHS itself – has not had a good long, expensive trial. And it is that original idea of 1946 that is obstructing his new idea, even though he thinks his second idea may save his first.

Perhaps that would be poetic justice. But the whole incident teaches a much more fundamental lesson. It is that the vast machine of the NHS will not yield to reasonable, civilised argument for reform that would disturb it – however beneficial the new idea might be for patients, doctors and everyone else.

And that brings me to the third view.

3. No case for all-embracing monopoly NHS ever

This is that there was *never* a case for an all-embracing NHS precisely for the reason that it would shut out or discourage new ideas – such as Lord Taylor's new one might be now. And that applied to Lord Taylor's main idea in the first place.

This conclusion points to the really damaging charge that can be made against everyone who thinks his idea so good that all other ideas must be shut out if it is to demonstrate how good it is.

We can never be certain that this is true of any idea. That is why no idea should be allowed to be exclusive. Every idea, however good it seems, should be tried in conditions where others can also be tried, as Lord Taylor's, 'alongside it'.

And that is the argument for a "market" for all kinds of ideas, systems, techniques, methods of paying for medical care. The very idea of "the market" is that no one idea is sacrosanct. The idea is that there shall be *no "final" solution* but that all ideas shall be tried out. The NHS is a "final solution" that has lasted longer than its more notorious namesake.

That is what is meant by arguing for competition in ideas between which people can choose.

*   *   *   *

This "market" approach – that there should be *no closed door to new thinking in health policy* – holds together the essays in this collection, even where the writers may differ. Their over-riding, common view is that they are pleading for an environment in which all ideas can be tried and the best can win – until something even better turns up.

These essays discuss the general principles of what has gone wrong with the NHS and what could be tried that looks – from commonsense or experience abroad – as if it might be better.

We try to show *why* reform is desirable. We indicate broadly *what* better system we should aim at. But we do not say *how* the reforms should be introduced.

There is no blue-print here. The NHS cannot be wound down, dismantled, or broken up by political action from outside. But that is not necessary, It is breaking up from inside because of weaknesses embodied in it – mainly the financing mechanism – that have been concealed by an endless procession of reorganisations, the latest in 1980.

The weakness can no longer be hidden. Doctors continue to leave the NHS – or Britain itself. Patients are going to doctors outside the NHS. New private services are emerging and expanding.

What now remains is to remove the obstacles to doctors and patients coming together, if they so wish, *outside* the NHS for better medical care than can be obtained inside it.

To ensure the removal of these obstructions, a better-informed public opinion – more sceptical of the eternal claims for the NHS, even angry with those who make them, and insistent on reform – is an essential. These essays should make the public sceptical, and angry, and insistent.

*   *   *   *

This preamble to the essays should justify the general title. The NHS has done the health of the people a "dis-service" because it has prevented the development of more spontaneous, organic, local, voluntary and *sensitive* medical services that would have grown up as incomes rose and medical science and technology advanced. If it were not for the *politically*-controlled NHS we should have seen new forms of medical organisation and financing that better reflected *consumer* preferences, requirements and circumstances. These lost opportunities of better medical care are the dis-service the NHS has done the people of Britain.

II
Better Medical Attention for All
– in the Midlands

Bernard Juby

MRCS Eng., LRCP London 1962, MRCGP 1969. Resigned from NHS 1966 and has practised privately. Member, National Federation of Self-Employed and Small Businesses. Chairman, West Midlands and Staffordshire Region, and a member of the National Insurance Sub-Committee.

Dr. Juby's patients are people from all social classes in a large Midland city. In 1965 he 'invited my patients to pay direct for medical care of the standard to which I had been trained.' He gives his patients more time with better equipment – and perhaps most fundamental, the assurance that if they are not satisfied they can easily go elsewhere.

THE National "Disease" Service (it is largely disease – rather than health – orientated) has done relatively little to help the human lot in health and welfare. Longer strides have been achieved in hygiene, shelter and nutrition to account for better basic health and longevity than the whole of the thirty-plus years since the inception of the NHS.

Good health is not a "basic right" to be provided by the State at all costs, especially when many of the nation's ills are self-inflicted. Without food, shelter and warmth Man would rapidly perish. Where are the cries of, 'Free Food, Free Heating and Free Homes?' Instead we get the emotive 'Free Health'.

NHS not providing good family doctoring

The concept of a "free" health service is now wearing thin as it becomes increasingly obvious to a tax-conscious public that the NHS is simply not delivering the goods. It is no use promising a free washing machine to all and sundry and then, when demand outstrips supply, either give a bar of soap and a wash-board or (more frequently) nothing at all: but that is the NHS in parts of Britain today.

Human nature is a fact of life. Unless we are forced against our will to become a race of Pavlovian salivants we will always be more ready and willing to spend money where we can see the direct result of that action benefitting ourselves or our immediate dependants. I am therefore now wholeheartedly in favour of private medical care, paid for *directly* (or through personal insurance) by the patient to the doctor. This would cut out the expensive governmental middle-man while at the same time allowing the patient to assess directly whether he or she was getting good value for money or not.

At present, unless they are already private patients, few people outside the medical profession know how much a bed in a hospital costs, the difference in value between a heart transplant and a hernia operation, or even the value of the drugs on a doctor's prescription. Individual costings should be made widely public at all times, so that value for money as well as the true cost of provision could be judged by the public and compared with costs in the private sector. The public have been spending some £50m in taxes *per day* on health and social security. Government's money does not come from gold mines underneath Downing Street or Whitehall. It comes from the pockets of taxpayers. Employment Secretary, James Prior, recently told radio listeners: 'There is no great pit in the back of Whitehall where we dig the money out.' Current needs and future requirements in Health Service spending (despite the announced cut-backs) will require even larger shovelfuls of that same money if the present NHS expectations continue to be met. It is *our* money and we should therefore be allowed more say in how it should be spent.

The people are turning away from the NHS

But the message is clearly filtering through. People are turning to alternative means of obtaining health care, either through self-education via organisations such as Weight-Watchers, Yoga and Keep Fit, or through private medicine (British United Provident Association, Private Patients Plan, screening clinics, etc.) in an attempt to fill the gaps either in time, availability or service that are glaringly apparent in the NHS.

In 1965 I decided to practice what I preached and invited my patients to pay me directly for my services. My practice is surrounded by large council housing estates.

To the south and to the north east are the prosperous dormitory towns of Solihull and Sutton Coldfield; nearby there is a mixture of owner-occupied housing (which has increased due to Council house sales), small shops and factories. It is thus a truly mixed suburban area, with the industry geared towards the motor car.

Medicine is a business

Despite altruistic motives and a certain degree of philanthopy, medicine is a business as well as an art. "A fair day's pay for a fair day's work" is as true now as it was in 1965. Before 1965 the arrangements for pay in our practice (after allowance for overheads) worked out at one pound per patient per year. Since the average patient consulted some five times in that year, the NHS were paying the equivalent of 20p (4 shillings) a time. Relatively speaking little has changed. To achieve a minimum income – regardless of services offered – most general practitioners had to carry lists of some 2500–3500 people. Taking an average of three thousand this meant some 15,000 consultations a year. If each took ten minutes some seven hours per day, every day, for 365 days per year has to be set aside in order to cope. The addition of time-consuming visits, lengthier problems, ante-natal clinics as well as holidays, days off (if any), special medicals and so on, meant that inadequate time to cope with current demand was and is a major cause of the dissatisfaction experienced on both sides of the medical consultation.

Furthermore, patients expecting the "five guineas worth" of care for 20p were going to be sadly disappointed. The problem was that they didn't know that 20p was all the State allowed – although they *did* know that it cost much, much more to have a service engineer call to unblock the drains, mend the television or call to fix the car *because they had to pay for it at the time.*

Phase 1 – annual pre-payment or item-of-service fees

I decided that a means had to be found whereby patients would get a better understanding of the true cost of medicine by similarly paying for it direct. Initially, since many were accustomed to "putting a bit away on the slate" or into sick-clubs, holiday clubs and the like, a scheme was devised whereby patients could pre-pay by weekly (subsequently found to be unpopular), monthly, quarterly, half-yearly and annual sums. The cost was calculated at the "price of a pint or a packet of fags" per person per week; the equivalent of some £6.00 to £8.00 a year. This sum was to cover drugs as well as my services and was a big improvement on NHS rates of pay, even allowing for the average 50p per prescription or £2.50 per person per year. There was also the option of item-of-service payments – the rates being 50p to £1.00 per surgery consultation and £1.00 to £2.00 per home visit with cost of drugs, special services, etc. extra.

Ds, Es and pensioners go private

Out of a total of 5,500 patients roughly one quarter opted to "go private". They included patients from all socio-economic classes from A to E almost in an exact proportion to the percentage of each class throughout the country. There were thus more class D and E than C2s and more class C2s than As and Bs. Surprisingly many "old age pensioners", clearly remembering the old pre-NHS days and wishing to return to them, opted to join the scheme. What was equally encouraging was that young married couples, spoon-fed on the Welfare State, contracted for private care in increasing numbers despite young families and probably heavy mortgage commitments. And all this despite the fact that anyone buying private medical care in Britain at present does so *in addition* to the large amounts they are paying in rates and taxes for the NHS.

Paying for medical attention

But what exactly are they paying for, especially when, as for education, etc., they are paying twice? First and foremost they are buying my time and my skills at a price they feel is a "fair" rate for the job. If they don't feel this is value for money they will not come again and go elsewhere. Most new patients consult a doctor as a result of a personal recommendation from a friend or business colleague. I am therefore rigidly controlled by market forces, unlike the NHS which pays up regardless of whether the end result is good, bad, indifferent or even rendered at all. They also enable me to buy equipment which I consider necessary for the practice of good medicine and which is used ultimately for their good. I am able to buy at a time when I consider it is required, rather than have to await a bureaucratic decision, regarding allocation of suitable funds.

As with all private patients, they pay in the knowledge that they will see the doctor of their choice; that any drugs required will be the best available for the job, reflecting also the best price of many available equivalents; they will have as much time allotted to them as is required for their problem, whether a mere five to ten minutes or an hour or more; and they will be seen at a time and day convenient to both parties.

While I can only offer my personal skills, I can do so without the thought of a waiting room full of patients awaiting attention in the "five–ten minute circus". Often under those circumstances a patient is also acutely aware that he is keeping the next one waiting; in his haste he fails to ask that important question or give that vital piece of information necessary to solve his problem. Above all he is paying in order to communicate at relative leisure; and, as in any professional contract, expects and has a right to my undivided attention and the guarantee that I will do my best within my ability.

Tailoring medicine to fit the patient

Increasingly many more doctors as well as patients are turning to an alternative to the NHS and are devising various schemes which are tailor-made to fit their circumstances and localities. There are of course snags and pitfalls, although the climate has changed radically since 1965 when a spate of doctors were resigning from the NHS for various reasons. Some emigrated; others gave up medicine altogether; some retired early; but many more set up their own private alternatives. The government of the day tried to crush them out by "bribing" doctors at much higher remuneration to move into areas thus "vacated" in order to set up direct competition. Despite the often lean first couple of years during which there is a heavy burden of tax liability from the previous "good" year, private practice providing general medical services flourishes and grows.

10

Phase II – full item-of-service

Many of the schemes are by monthly payment. While it may eventually lead to a full item-of-service method of payment, any scheme which is a small scale version of the NHS still removes the true cost from the patient. Unless there is an inbuilt 'nominal' fee at each consultation, the selfish, neurotic and dependents become frequent visitors as there is no limit to the number of attendances one could ask. The overall pattern therefore developed over the years into a full item-of-service type of payment as the only true and "fair" way of remuneration for work done. This is the method of payment frequently requested by the medical profession since 1948 but not yet fully available in the NHS.

It may be that preventive medicine, public health, accident and emergency work could be best supplied by the State via a much slimmer NHS. The remaining health care should be hived off to the market place, where the true cost (and hence appreciation) of medical care can become apparent to all. Trade union members are not averse to "going private". They often put up the money to enable another member of the family or a relative to do likewise. With government taking care of the "poor" by subsidies (i.e. a reverse income tax) and encouraging the rest by income tax allowances, there is no reason why the populace as a whole should not be able to afford it.

My experiences over the past fourteen years prove that the public *is* ready and willing. It only requires the courage of government to release the brakes and let free the juggernaught of private enterprise in the provision of health care.

III
Better Medical Attention for All
– In Southern England

Patrick Wood

Qualified at St. Bartholomews in 1944 and served for five years in the RAMC. Entered private general practice in Suffolk in 1950. In 1960 awarded one of the first Nuffield Travelling Fellowships for GPs and studied for six months in America. He has been Chairman of The Fellowship for Freedom in Medicine since 1967.

A second family doctor, Dr Patrick Wood, has only private patients in Suffolk – from the elderly poor, through factory workers and trades people to people in management and the professions. He describes private family doctoring, with its unique mutual confidence and trust between doctor and patient, as a cheap *service that could be available for all. He argues that the central fault of the NHS is its (indirect) method of payment: by the patient in taxes and then by the government to doctors.*

THE 47 year old telephonist developed a swollen gland in her neck. Two weeks later her throat became sore and she went to the Health Centre. She was seen by Dr A who said it was an infection and treated her with antibiotics. There was no improvement, so she went back to the Health Centre and was seen by Dr B. He prescribed a different antibiotic. Her symptoms persisted so she returned and succeeded in seeing Dr A. He advised a longer course of antibiotics. When this course was completed her throat was more sore and the gland bigger. By now very worried she returned to the Health Centre. She couldn't see Dr A or Dr B so was seen by Dr C, who prescribed yet more antibiotics. Not surprisingly the telephonist lost all confidence. She wasn't any better; she felt none of the doctors was responsible for her. Although of modest means she decided the next day to see a private doctor. The doctor examined her and found a hard gland in her neck. When she opened her mouth he could see on the back wall of her throat a large malignant ulcer. No instruments were required for this examination. She had cancer, and a cancer which had spread into her glands. A throat specialist saw her the next day and confirmed the diagnosis. In his letter to the private doctor the specialist wrote 'the way this patient has been handled is a terrible indictment of Health Centre medicine'. She was treated under the NHS promptly and effectively from that moment on.

Political fashion

This case is a true horror story. One cannot argue from the particular to the general, but it is not necessarily an advantage to be treated by several different doctors. Health Centres, although politically fashionable, do not always encourage the highest standards of medicine. They have their virtues and their vices. Perhaps I am cynical in believing that most of their virtues relate to the convenience of the doctors and staff who run them, and most of their vices affect the patients.

Medical care in general practice is a personal and private matter. Patients want to get to know their doctor, to build up a trust in him, to feel they can rely on him when they are ill. They want their doctor to "care". There is nothing worse for the patient than an off-hand doctor who hasn't time to listen, who seems too busy to make more than a cursory examination, if any, and who is writing a prescription within a minute or two of the patient walking into the room.

As doctors, we sometimes blame the media for enlarging on the dangers of drugs, but it is difficult for patients to have confidence in treatment ordered by their doctor if he seems to use the prescription as a method of cutting short the consultation rather than as a genuine healing weapon.

Passengers survive as inefficient doctors in the NHS

Why is it that in the last thirty years, when medicine has made spectacular advances in the physician's effectiveness in dealing with many of the commonest illnesses, that the status of the family doctor has diminished? He has therapies available to him to deal with acute infections, rheumatism, stomach ulcers, heart failure, skin diseases and the whole gamut of psychological illness which make him a giant compared to the pygmy figure of the pre-war doctor. Yet, far from being a man of stature, he is now only sometimes respected, and rarely loved. Is this decline a failure of the doctors, or of the system?

As in any other profession, doctors can be divided into the good, the bad, and the average. I believe good doctors do good work under whatever system of medicine they are functioning. It makes little difference to their efficiency whether they are paid by capitation fee or on an item-of-service basis as are solicitors, accountants, etc. They may not like the system but they overcome its faults.

Bad doctors do bad work under whatever system of medicine they are functioning, but it is very much *easier* for them to earn a comfortable living paid by capitation fee (as in the NHS) than if they were exposed to market forces and competition. There are passengers in NHS general practice who would not survive three months in the hard world outside.

It is to the great bulk of average doctors that we must look to see if thirty years of the NHS have provided a system which maintains morale, which encourages good work and effort, and which discourages slackness, apathy and intolerance. For the life of a GP is very hard; to work permanently in an environment of ill-health, suffering, and mental and emotional disease is inevitably arduous. The doctor has to give encouragement, good cheer, and reassurance, and this constant giving exhausts his resources. In addition to this he carries a weight of daily responsibility – his patient with constipation may have cancer of the bowel, the man who thinks he has indigestion may have coronary heart disease, the woman with depression may commit suicide. The potential for daily disaster is limitless, and it is the awareness of this danger, allied to the need for sensitivity and real understanding, that becomes such a strain over the years.

If you combine these factors with the long working hours, the night calls, the importance of acting effectively in dealing with the many crises of acute mental and physical disease in which individuals and whole families face sudden peril and unhappiness, then even the most unimaginative person may realise that to be a family doctor can never be easy and, at times, can be the most difficult job in the world. That it can be one of the most rewarding is equally true. Most doctors get back from their patients more than they give, and they are genuinely revitalised by their gratitude, affection and love.

But if the doctor's morale is low, if he is tired, disillusioned and cynical, he gives out little to his patients and gets little back. Before long his patients become his enemy.

The NHS method of payment is wrong

Morale is an intangible quality; it depends on work satisfaction and remuneration to a substantial extent. Doctors are ordinary men and women with families to bring up, houses and cars to buy, and holidays to enjoy. They train for many years to study the intricacies of an ever-expanding scientific discipline and then apply their knowledge to all the vagaries of human nature. They deserve to be "adequately" paid. The reader may have some sympathy with this view but feel that the method of remuneration of his GP is of little concern. I strongly disagree, because the NHS *method* of payment is one of its fundamental weaknesses.

The GP is paid partly by salary and partly by capitation fees, with other minor additions. Seniority is recognised, merit is not. The capitation fee (so much per head for each patient registered with the doctor) is paid exactly the same whether he is seen not once in a year or a hundred times. If the doctor sees his patient only once or twice a year, the capitation fee is a reasonable return for his work. If he attends him many times the payment is derisory.

This curious method of payment is thus a disincentive to see the same patient repeatedly. A doctor's life is so demanding that to manage without incentives must be extremely difficult. He is trained to deal with serious illness in the patient's home and could derive "work satisfaction" from doing so, but this involves heavy responsibility and much time. It is so much easier to refer a patient who requires investigation to a hospital consultant, so much easier to admit to hospital all patients who are acutely ill rather than visit them repeatedly at home. Many patients who could be dealt with in the inexpensive home sector of medicine are thus pushed into costly hospital care entirely due to the way the GP is paid.

Patients are unwanted

The trouble goes even deeper. Patients who require a lot of care and attention are not only uneconomic but also unwanted. The old and the chronic sick, the people who most need good GP care, are refused by some doctors who prefer a large list of healthy patients requiring the minimum of attention.

Many good doctors in the NHS provide devoted care without any financial incentive. But the capitation-fee system is not a sensible way of getting the best out of the bulk of the profession.

The method of remuneration is not the only reason for low morale. A major factor is that the GP is faced with a service free at the time of use. Here we are at the bedrock of the problems the NHS has created, and it is necessary to stand back to get a clearer perspective. Emotion and political dogma have clouded this issue for too long: even after thirty years, entrenched positions are still held by opposing sides fighting a ghostly war in which reality was the earliest casualty.

NHS rations by time

The ideal is of a free-at-the-time service with equal access to medical care for all. Most people would agree philosophically that the best possible medical care for all should be available regardless of the ability of the individual to pay. It is only when you face economic reality that you realise this ideal is a mirage. Medical care has to be paid for. In general practice it is reasonably cheap; in hospital care, with all the sophisticated apparatus and highly trained staff to use it, it is expensive. Either you pay for your medical care yourself directly or through insurance, or you pay the State to provide it for you. If you *cannot* pay, the State *must*.

In post-war Britain the people decided to ask the state to provide a medical service for them. At the time they did not realise it must cost them more; because there was no direct consumer control, wastage and extravagance were inevitable, and they had to finance a huge bureaucracy to administer the service. Nor did they realise they would have to make sacrifices. They did not foresee that freedom of choice in medical care, the right to see your own doctor or specialist, would diminish in a nationalised service.

Above all, and this was the cardinal error, they did not understand that, if you provide such an essential and valuable service free at the time of use, you create unlimited demand. Everyone understands that our resources in doctors, hospitals and equipment are finite and restricted. The only way finite resources can cope with

16

unlimited demand is by imposing a barrier between doctor and patient – the barrier of time. The long delays in obtaining treatment, the queues in the surgery, the 750,000 or more on hospital waiting lists, are all an essential, permanent, and in-built part of the NHS system. Waiting lists are not just statistics, they are ill people suffering pain and disability. (The significance of waiting for the NHS is analysed by Profesor Cotton Lindsay in Essay VIII—Ed.) They are not a theoretical conception which can be debated. Their existence is a potent criticism of the human cost of the NHS.

"Equal" access to deteriorating service

This is not the only cost. Thirty years' experience has shown us that a tax-financed service can *never* raise enough money to provide modern well-equipped hospitals and a well-paid and satisfied staff. Financial stringency leads to loss of morale, to defensive trade unionism, and to a reduction in goodwill. Vocation has been destroyed in the "caring" professions to a dangerous and frightening extent. We are paying a heavy price for the essentially socialist ideal – or myth – of a "free" service.

What is the good of equal access to medical care if it has deteriorated? – If there is not enough finance to build hospitals and run them properly? – If doctors and staff are discontented and disillusioned? Equality of access means little to the patient who waits 2 to 3 hours to see his doctor in the surgery and then has a couple of minutes: too little time to explain his symptoms or be properly examined. Equality of access means little to the 70-year-old in pain day and night who has to wait two years or more for a hip replacement.

Equality for the trivial and the serious

It is against this background that the GP has to cope with a service free at the time of use. His most obvious problem is that open access to all allows the trivial equal priority with serious illness. He has to defend himself from spending as much time on a patient with a pimple on her face as the patient with cancer. Some patients are considerate, some are not; some make totally unreasonable demands on his services. Some patients feel at a disadvantage because the consultation is free, and the sense of obligation can make them prickly and aggressive. Others are determined to get their "rights" and to exploit a free service to the full. There seems little doubt that a free-at-the-time service devalues the doctor, and that the nominal prescription charge (even at £1.00) misleads the public about the real cost of drugs and leads to extravagances, waste and misuse.

Counterbalancing these factors is the natural goodwill in all patients for doctors and nurses who care for them in time of illness. I have often heard it said "I am truly grateful to the NHS". But when questioned it becomes clear that their gratitude is for their doctor, nurse or hospital. It is rarely remembered that the NHS is only a system of medical care. Doctors, nurses and hospitals were doing their jobs long before the NHS was created. And they will continue to do so long after its demise.

The NHS is misconceived and fundamentally unsound. The principle of equal access to medical care for all regardless of means, although fine in theory cannot work in practice. The NHS is not designed to get the best out of the average GP because it lacks incentive, lowers morale, and reduces work satisfaction.

The Alternative: Private practice for all

There is no case for a totally nationalised service. The State does not have to own the hospitals or employ all the doctors and nurses. Medical staff work much better for their patients than for the State. Hospitals can be run much more efficiently locally than centrally.

If we accept that the aim is that all should have medical care available to them whatever their means, it is up to the State to ensure that the poor, the chronic sick and the handicapped are its responsibility, for they cannot fend for themselves. The resources of the State should be concentrated in these areas. The rest of the community should be encouraged to pay for themselves.

Private practice is the natural relationship of doctor to patient with a fee charged for each item of service. General practice is still a comparatively inexpensive form of medical care. It is a delusion to think that private practice is only for the wealthy. Naturally in opulent areas like the West End of London some doctors charge high fees, but scattered over Britain there is private "catering" for all income groups and all social classes.

My family doctor service

In our own practice we have genuinely poor elderly patients living on small fixed incomes who are hard hit by inflation. Even a few on supplementary benefit prefer to spend on private care despite the availability of a "free" service. We have self-employed craftsmen and tradesmen who value highly the doctors' efforts to get them back to work quickly, and increasing numbers of manual and semi-skilled workers from the factory floor. These men have good incomes and low expenses, and are not content to spend their surplus money entirely on holidays, smoking, and so on. At the other end of the scale we have an occasional millionaire and many from the professional and managerial classes.

The satisfied patient soon wants his wife and children to be treated by the doctor who wins his confidence, and we have looked after the same families for many years. We are on Christian name terms with most of our patients.

We have deliberately pitched our charges on the low side of average in order to give our practice as wide and stable a base as possible. This policy has stood us in good stead in the inflationary crisis of the last six years. We charge less for a home visit than would a plumber or electrician. Although it may seem paradoxical that a patient in heart failure and threatened with death can be treated for less than it takes to service a washing machine, the reason is simple. Household appliances can be thrown away and replaced when they are uneconomic, patients cannot. The more worn out and unhealthy a patient becomes, the more care he requires. The costing of medical treatment needs a generous leaven of compassion.

After thirty years in private practice, I have no doubt that patients are prepared to spend far more money directly on medical care than they would ever contribute through taxation. They value their health and are prepared to make financial sacrifices for it.

The private doctor is at present in competition with a "free" service. His patients have to pay his fees and the full cost of drugs prescribed. In order to compete effectively the doctor has to give that most valuable of commodities: time. He cannot *afford not* to listen to his patients' symptoms, or fail to carry out a thorough examination. As a result of the reassurance patients feel when they are looked after in this way, they often do not require any medicine at all. If they do, it has to be prescribed with considerable thought about the cost. Economy in prescribing is an important consideration for the private doctor, if not his NHS counterpart. Some patients, whose essential drugs are too costly, are lost to private care.

A bond, not a barrier

It has been argued that the professional fee is a barrier and may prevent the patient seeking advice early in the course of an illness. I have found very little evidence to support this contention. The fee is a bond, not a barrier. The paying patient employs the doctor's services. Payment gives the patient status and authority and makes him an *equal partner* in the consultation. (In NHS practice the balance of power unduly favours the doctor.) The close relationship between private doctor and patient based on mutual understanding and affection is a powerful force in maintaining the doctor's morale under stress. If the patient is demanding, or late for an appointment, or inconsiderate in requesting an unnecessary visit, the doctor can adjust his fee. This saves much of the frustration experienced by NHS doctors.

Charging by item-of-service is flexible; it can cover any eventuality, and the doctor feels he is being paid for the work he does. This encourages him to tackle serious illness in the patient's home, and to investigate complex conditions himself rather than overload the hospital. It has been argued by the opponents of item-of-service charges that they create much book-work. I work in a partnership of two doctors employing one secretary who does telephone answering during office hours, much of the dispensing, and all the book-work and accounts.

Everyone could have private family doctoring

If the State were to concentrate its resources on the poor, the handicapped and the chronic sick, these groups could be subsidised to obtain private medical treatment on the same terms as their more fortunate brothers. When the State spends money it must control and regulate: clearly some bureaucracy is inevitable. Item-of-service payments must be more complex than salary and capitation fees to administer, but the micro-processor revolution will simplify and speed up office work.

Although insurance is important in medical care, its role lies far more in the costly hospital sector than in general practice. The demand for medical care in general practice is largely subjective. The only way to contain limitless demand is for the patient himself to pay a substantial part of the fee.

If he pays a premium which entitles him to 100 per cent reimbursement, this is the surest way to send medical costs sky high. (Further discussed by Hugh Elwell in Essay XVIII—Ed.). I do not believe that insurance in general practice should cover more than 50 per cent of the cost. (I exclude the State subsidised patients from this limit.)

If private practice were to replace NHS care in general practice, the State would have to assist those patients requiring expensive or long-term therapy.

We have had over thirty years of the great NHS experiment. We can only make progress by going back. If we can use all that is good in private practice for the benefit of the whole community, and especially for people most in need, for the sake of both doctor and patient we must dismantle an NHS which has become incompetent, uncaring and unloved.

IV
Better Health Care for All
– in the North East

John Noble

John Noble is a general practitioner in Northumberland. He is a Member of the BMA Council and of its General Medical Services Committee. He has served on numerous committees and written extensively about General Practice in the National Health Service. He served on the government Working Party on General Practice and was co-author of the Northumberland Local Medical Council's paper "An expanding remit for General Practice".

Introduction

This essay explores an expanding role for general practice based on Charter 2 proposals of the Northumberland Local Medical Committee, 1978. The doctor will provide a wider range of personal services for fewer patients, with modern equipment and facilities. The general practitioner will carry out preventive and curative medicine at all ages, and perform much of the routine work now done by consultant, and particularly non-consultant, staff in hospitals and specialist clinics. Such a system would use the skills and foster the vocational aspirations of doctors, providing comprehensive patient care. The relative costs of primary and hospital care should make the proposition attractive to Government. Prompt and comprehensive care at the point of initial contact would appeal to the patient.

The frustrations and limitations of the NHS family doctor

The general practitioner, the traditional approach of the British to medical care, contracts to provide what are called necessary and appropriate medical services to the patients who join his list. Because of the allocation scheme, which empowers the Minister to place any patient without a doctor on a general practitioner's list, the NHS family doctors take over the statutory duty of the Government to provide personal medical care to every citizen with 24-hour cover for the vast majority of clinical incidents in the population from beginning to end.

The contract relates to availability, the work load is dictated by demand. In order to accommodate this, the time for each patient is compressed on an average to five minutes, efficiency is diminished and the development of general practice is impeded. As a result, far too many patients are referred to hospital, and then held in the Out-Patients Department where they should be (but are usually not) dealt with by the general practitioner. Family doctors are becoming increasingly frustrated by this pattern of medical care. And a discerning public is showing disenchantment at the failure of the NHS to provide the medical care they demand, as evidenced by complaints about appointment systems and lengthy hospital waiting lists, and the emergence in places of the 24 hour private service.

The challenge: aims

It is in the interests of good quality personal medical care that general practitioners expand their role in providing personal services to their patients, using their skills to the full. If this policy were adopted, medical treatment, and the efficiency and vocational satisfaction of doctors would be revolutionised, especially in the connurbations where general practice is commonly acknowledged to be at a low ebb. General practitioners would revive their pride in work well done and provide a secure basis for health care. Only in this way can individual patient care be improved.

The description of general practice by an EEC Working Party in 1975 is generally acceptable (although it does not define *quality* without which it is impossible to measure efficacy or *patient* satisfaction):

> The general practitioner is a licensed medical graduate, who gives personal, primary and continuing care to individuals, families and a practice population, irrespective of age, sex and illness. It is the synthesis of those functions which is unique. He will attend his patients in his consulting room and in their homes and sometimes in a clinic or a hospital. His aim is to make early diagnosis. He will include and integrate physical, psychological and social factors in his considerations about health and

illness. This will be expressed in the care of patients. He will make an initial decision about every problem presented to him as a doctor. He will undertake the continuing management of his patients with chronic, recurrent or terminal illness. Prolonged contact means he can use repeated opportunities to gather information at a pace appropriate to each patient and build up a relationship of trust which he can use professionally. He will practise in co-operation with other colleagues, medical and non-medical. He will know how and when to intervene through treatment, prevention and education to promote the health of his patients and their families. He will recognise that he also has a professional responsibility to the community.

The vocational status of the general practitioner is thus:

i. He is clinically responsible for the continuing medical care of his patients, diffused so that with adequate facilities, time and help he should be able to diagnose and treat all conditions which do not require highly specialised consultant opinion, or institutional investigation and treatment. This reform could be achieved by a minor reorientation of resources, manpower and facilities, but it would require sharper incentives than in the NHS.

ii. The general practitioner, legally responsible for the patients, must be leader of the primary care team and should be trained as such, especially in his relationship with the other elements of the team, their aspirations and their professional ethics.

iii. The general practitioner should have adequate time to fulfil his responsibility to deal with curative and preventive medicine in the home and to advise his patients on the maintenance of their health and the use of medicines.

iv. It is not the duty of doctors to prop up ailing health services by rushed work which leads to lowering standards. This must cease.

The framework of general practice

i. How would these concepts work in practice? The family doctors would provide comprehensive diagnostic and therapeutic care to the patient, limited only by their skills, to include preventive medicine and surveillance to patients of all ages, paediatric and geriatric screening. Since most doctors now have adequate premises the medical care should include minor operative procedures, manipulation, intra-articular therapy, cardiograph and indeed any investigative or other activity which can be carried out as well, more personally and promptly, in the family doctor's premises. Some general practitioners possess special skills. They are permitted to spend five sessions per week in hospital deploying them. It would be much better, in appropriate cases, if they used them at the patient's point of contact.

ii. Some 6000 to 8000 additional general practitioners would counter-balance a reduction in the total of hospital doctors. The general practitioner's Terms of Service would need revision in line with the new arrangement, but the most important element would be a re-orientation of his income to recognise his wider responsibility and provide incentives for them to be carried out, but an increasingly aware public, provoking a degree of clinical competition would introduce a degree of "consumer audit".

Ancillary elements

i. *Premises*

In the NHS the arrangements for provision of premises operate favourably for doctors who practice from Health Centres and adversely against those in private premises. The arrangements through the cost rent, improvement grant schemes and general practice finance corporation should be reformed to give the doctor with private premises equal opportunities. The cost of more equipment would have to be recognised in assessing the overall terms.

ii. *Ancillary Staff: direct reimbursement?*

Financial curbs and the failure due to the institutional orientation of health authorities in some areas, to recognise the importance of the community nursing and health visiting services and their integration with general practice must be corrected. If these services continue to suffer disproportionally as a result of NHS cuts, it may be necessary for such staff to be employed through the direct reimbursement scheme for general practice expenses. Financial control would be maintained as the scheme reimburses only up to 70 per cent of costs.

Extra services would also be required in the Family Doctors' premises, including physiotherapy, occupational therapy and social work. General practice recording should be brought up to date: the medical record conceived in 1911 or even before is inadequate for modern needs.

Practice Management

This has become a sophisticated element of good general practice and is integral to smooth and efficient running of a family doctor unit, the satisfaction of the patients and the vocational fulfilment of the doctors. Practice managers of high quality are emerging. But it is essential that one of a group of general practitioners, or each in turn, should supervise the management and translating practice policy into operational terms. Vocational training should prepare the doctor for this task.

Study time

Time for study and refreshment of learning is essential and should be an inseparable part of the working day. It must be carefully planned and individuals encouraged to implement their own ideas. Such activities must be adequately financed and remunerated either through basic fees or directly from the patient to each item of service.

Is comprehensive care in general practice possible?

In spite of the NHS system of remuneration, which does little or nothing to encourage good medicine, many practices provide some or part of the services described, but to do so must reduce their lists, and remuneration, to create the necessary time. There are also private general practitioners who provide such a service at modest cost, and they are not all in the so-called more prosperous areas.

Changes in the method of remuneration of family doctors to create incentives could produce changes rapidly. Immunisation has returned to family medicine, so has ante-natal care and contraception. Cervical cytology payments, though small, are an example of screening. All are paid by fees for each item of service.

The metamorphosis would occur in the service provided in general practice if pay was orientated to service rather than availability. Extra cash would be required for the additional doctors but the reduced load on the hospitals and other institutions would save money and release personnel. Many general practitioners working part-time in hospital would return to a more complete and satisfying primary care. In the same way a remunerative differential for doctors who, either individually or in small groups, provide their own out-of-hours and emergency services, would encourage personal care, and deputising services would be less attractive.

Doctor to remain independent

The general practitioner should retain his status as an independent contractor. This is a major safeguard for the trust which a patient can have in his doctor and in the confidentiality of the consultation. The vast majority of general practitioners understand and believe this proposition and turn to consider a salaried status only out of frustration with the NHS. The objective is for each doctor to be responsible for his own patients.

Paying for the new service

Many general practitioners are opposed to charging patients at the time of use of the service. They are also concerned that a vast increase of item-of-service payments would cause unnecessary form filling, but the latter could be controlled by common sense and disciplining of bureaucracy.

Ensuring provision

Doctors would require to be convinced that their efforts were recognised by proportionate remuneration if the better service were provided. There is nothing wrong with a true productivity deal. The public would wish to know they would get improved medical care. A degree of clinical competition would be their best assurance. Yet medical men vary in capacity and dedication, and audit would be essential. There would be two clear elements, the professionals dealing with clinical matters and an audit to ensure that work done was required, and had been performed.

Finance

Because the National Health Service is not properly item costed the economics of the shift to full care at the point of contact are difficult to assess but, if it costs around £5 to see a general practitioner, £20 to enter a casualty department and £50 if a procedure is performed, the indication is clear.

Finally, and these are the writer's views, as elsewhere with financial pressures operating, private general practice could develop for the very reasons given above, providing efficient, relatively cheap and complete care. This would create two tiers of care which I believe would be unacceptable and unnecessary.

The answer is a shift to the community, where treatment could be cheaper, prompt and more personal. If there is not enough money and energy to do even this, then it is time the NHS ceased to be a monolith the State cannot afford and become a mixed economy like the rest of society.

V

Hospitals are for Patients

John Cozens-Hardy

FRCS – Consultant Orthopaedic Surgeon, North Birmingham District, based on Good Hope Hospital, Sutton Coldfield (appointed 1965). Born in Norwich 1922. Medical training Oxford and St. Bartholomew's Hospital. Qualified 1946, the year of the NHS Act. More or less abandoned medicine for the Royal Navy 1947–1953.

A consultant orthopaedic surgeon in Birmingham, Mr Cozens-Hardy, explains his frustrations in the NHS. Because it cannot raise enough funds in taxes, he has to tell patients requiring hip replacements to wait four to five years. He is gently angry at hospitals which seem to run more for the staff than for the patients. His "cri de coeur" goes to the root of the trouble: 'What does it matter where the money comes from as long as it comes?' It expresses the anguish of doctors concerned more with treating disease than with the egalitarian obsessions of politicians who confine "the money" for medical care to taxes.

A HAPPY ship is an efficient ship. If I have got it the wrong way round, it does not matter – one is the result of the other, either way. For every voyage a ship is entire and has a destination, known to all on board. The captain and the crew get her there.

In an efficient and, therefore, happy hospital service an orthopaedic surgeon, for example, would get on with the job, doing what he is trained and paid to do and enjoys doing (yes, the job itself is rewarding, not soul-destroying). Indeed, the *only* function of a hospital service is to provide the setting in which professionals can get on with their job.

This poses three questions: What is this job? What about patients? Is the only function of a health service to secure gainful employment for all those of whom an orthopaedic surgeon is but an example and for all those required to provide the setting in which all front-line workers can get on with the job? These are not three questions but one. There is only one answer to all three. Happiness and efficiency in a ship are two sides of the same coin. The doctor (and all those whom in this argument he represents) and the patient are two sides of the same coin. They cannot, functionally, be separated. If there are factors that succeed in separating them, we can switch metaphors back again and say that the ship loses its way. Abandon ship.

Hospitals for patients, not for staff

In 1979, before the publication of *The Times* ceased, there was for about a week a correspondence which became headed, "Hospital for Patients". The function of a hospital has been largely lost to view; we need to be reminded almost as if it were a novel idea, what hospitals are for. It is not only the total outsider who might be startled, annoyed or brought to his senses by this suggestion: *for a change, let us have some hospitals for patients.*

It is difficult to proceed without giving the impression of being partisan. Accusations and counter-accusations of sectarianism indicate the first crack in the coin. Split apart its two sides and the service becomes a market place of interested parties – parties motivated by self-interest, parties disinterested in the patient.

What are the factors which have brought about this breach? One for sure is the sheer size, the sheer unmanageable bulk of the monolith, so that attempts to manage it are confounded and compounded and become increasingly insatiable. Two centuries ago Lord Chancellor Thurlow asked how anyone could expect a corporation to have a conscience when it had neither a soul to be damned nor a body to be kicked. Yet only a corporate conscience can preserve the coin. The NHS cannot have a conscience. If it ever had one – and some of us would like to think it had – it has lost it. Even if important people recognise this fact, are we not too off-course to find it?

In the NHS we are now queuing up – and not always quietly – for an increased wage. Is this in exchange for our souls? Hospitals provide jobs, jobs provide wages. So far in this country, on the whole, doctors have security of tenure. Established in our hospitals and in practice we are safe. The NHS has become so embroiled in labour and the welfare state that pressure is diverted from where it should be maintained – from the provision of what is best for the *patient* – to the preservation of *jobs*. Who, at this stage and in this set-up, can blame anyone?

Job creation for superfluous staff?

Most of us who work in hospital could each name perhaps half a dozen people who are superfluous and may even be harmful. This might seem a cruel observation; taken a little further it would be like standing by as a person was deprived of his livelihood. But these considerations would not arise if the NHS had not lost its way.

Patients are citizens and tax-payers, fully paid up members of the State. It is estimated that in 1978 each citizen of England and Wales, man, woman and child, contributed on average £141 to the NHS (that is, apart from the Social Services) or each family of four, £564. But can the breadwinner of such a family, the tax-payer, see where his money has gone? Does he have any say in how it is spent, or redress when it becomes clear it has been mis-spent? Whom can he identify as accountable when he is cheated of the benefits assured indelibly in the Statute Book?

For an annual subscription of £290 one Provident Association undertakes to provide a 60-year-old man, his wife and family with comprehensive health care. Those tax-payers (compulsory) who also subscribe (voluntarily) to such an association will usually, when needing treatment, choose the cover of the latter because care by the organisation to which they are compelled to contribute has in many areas become so bad. Therefore, they pay two subscriptions. Most tax-payers by upbringing rely on the State for health care but may find that when, emergencies apart, the need for treatment strikes them, the relief to which they are entitled is not forthcoming. They have paid their penny but are denied their choice. If they cannot find money for treatment outside they are trapped and become prisoners of their increasing pain and disability. (Pain is par excellence the sympton of the *orthopaedic* patient.) There is no escape for them. If they do find the money, and escape, they will be paying twice. The State has then both failed them and embezzled their contribution.

NHS hospitals deteriorate; private hospitals boom

Provident Associations are happy, and so are many doctors. NHS hospitals have deteriorated so much that there is a boom in private medicine with new hospitals and extensions to existing ones being built. A mood of congratulation prevails among the developers. People, they say, are being set free and choosing. They are choosing, increasingly, treatment outside the State. And they are usually well pleased with their choice.

But what about those who cannot afford to quit the ship? One should not have to ask. They are the very ones, who, as a group, by being well cared for, should have "disappeared" in the NHS, but it is they above all others whose tragedy the NHS has exposed. Beveridge and Bevan were miles out on their assumptions. TB and poliomyelitis were disappearing before 1948. Since then prevention and the spread of welfare has not, across the board, eliminated disease and steadily reduced the burden on the tax-payer. Surgical lists seem to be as full of malignant disease as they ever were. In my own case trauma and destructive joint disease – real suffering and real disability – outstrip what we can provide. Most Coronary Care units and Intensive Treatment Units are always busy.

I can speak only for my own patients, but I can speak for them as a group better than can anyone else. I am one among six hundred Consultant Orthopaedic Surgeons in the UK and at the jobbing end of the fraternity. There are four of us at the hospital where I work. Our patients suffer more than do those of many other districts because funds ran out and our hospital was never completed.

Four to five years for hip replacements

When, at the request of her GP, I see a new patient in one of my two weekly outpatient clinics, she may already have been waiting a year. She has had, let us say, three years of increasing pain and lameness from destructive arthritis of a hip. When the pain began to stop her sleeping, she went to see her doctor. Initially, drugs and physiotherapy helped a bit. I tell her that only an operation can restore her to most of what she could do and enjoy three years ago. She accepts; so I tell her I will put her name on the waiting list. She asks how long it will be before she comes in. I should, if she were to receive what she had paid for or what had been paid for on her behalf, be able to say four or five months (and that for some patients would be cruel news indeed). But what I have to answer is that it won't be four or five months, but four or five years or more.

The third rate is accepted as normal

Why don't these citizens, cheated of their right, march on Westminster? Firstly, of course, because it wouldn't occur to them to do so. Very few even approach their elected representatives in Parliament (to the relief of administrators). We have reached the point where the third rate is accepted as normal and something to be put up with. By the attrition of many years the patient can only shrug and say 'what's the use?' They are, therefore, secondly, a tiny and silent minority, and the provision of funds for the only resources which would bring them relief is controlled and prevented by politicians and by government that have other things to think about and other claims on its funds. This tiny minority carries no weight.

In his Edwin Stevens Lecture for the Laity in June 1979 the US Ambassador to Britain spoke of his admiration (yes, 'to the point of envy') for any society which can truly say that it has achieved non-discriminatory access to health care for all its citizens. Can we say that? Leaving aside falling standards and closer scrutiny of the *quality* of health care, we can only say that we already have a steady increase in rationing by queue and, therefore, discrimination. And who but politicians currently decide which queues shall be allowed to grow longer, and thus dictate which diseases or which sections of the community shall be treated?

In the Queens Bench Division in January 1979, after a hearing lasting five days, the learned judge found that the Secretary of State for Social Services had not failed in his statutory duty to provide what was necessary to bring relief to four patients of mine. He had every sympathy, he said, with what they had suffered and were suffering. It was all very regrettable.

Poor Mr Ennals, poor Barbara Castle, poor Mr Crossman, poor all of them, they had all tried so hard, but they just had not got the money. The Respondents (the Department of Health and Social Security, the Regional Health Authority and the Area Health Authority) had done all in their power, and now as an earnest of their concern we had the Resources Allocation Working Party. What more could the patients ask? All this Counsel for the Respondents took two whole days to say, reading out loud, word for word, most of RAWP's first report. In this he was assisted by frequent rests and glasses of water, and by his Junior. An Appeal was heard in March 1980 – and dismissed.

The NHS: "no funds" – a failure in political persuasion

So the problem is:– *no funds*. How, after all these years in which we have watched the steady growth of demand and the increasing restraints on supply (the former now almost unlimited and the latter cut back) has Government failed to persuade the British people that they can no longer have a NHS as it was originally conceived and launched? Is this connundrum related to the fact, for example, that an increase in prescription charges is so very newsworthy and always makes the headlines? Do politicians tremble? Are governments afraid? Are we so indoctrinated? Have we lost altogether our wizardry for the pragmatic solution for which we were once so famous? The NHS worked at first and most of us in hospitals were proud of it. That was fifteen years ago. *Is it working now?*

What does it matter where the money comes from as long as it comes? Why the obsession for the only source from which it so obviously is *not* coming – the Chancellor's General Taxation Fund? In September 1979 the Commissioners who took over the Lambeth, Southwark and Lewisham Area Health Authority "discovered" that its financial plight – and the plight of the rest of the Health Service – is far graver than has yet been admitted. Admitted by whom? In those who should have admitted it, whoever they were, but apparently did not, we have the emperor and his clothes. It is astonishing – frightening – that a fact of daily life that has been known to so many for so long should be suddenly presented as a discovery, let alone a discovery to make headlines – "*Inflation traps Authority*".

At a conference of the National Association of Health Authorities in September the Health Minister, having dismissed 'as a nonsense' accusations that the Government wanted to alter the NHS radically, went on to say that 'we want a vital flexible National Health Service which is available to everyone'. Who doesn't, and how in the name of all reasonable men and responsible citizens do they think they will get one without the other? Of whom, in the name of all suffering patients cheated of relief, is the Government so *afraid* that a key spokesman has to *squeak* like that?

Some patients and doctors will escape: the rest will be the victims

If Government cannot govern because the government of our country is no longer in its hands, we shall see the present trend accelerate. That is perhaps what this Government and its adherents are really after: two health services. Many patients and members of the health professions will escape from the worse to the better, and those patients who cannot take this route will be the remnants of a noble experiment which finally failed. Those on the inside, who took an active part in the experiment and, working on the shop floor, watched the failure as it remorselessly overtook them, did not at first give up hope. But now many of us are overcome by helplessness and despair, and are floundering with our patients in a quagmire which almost shapeless shapes stir from time to time. These spectres seem to have names and so too the spoons they use: Willink, Salmon, Joseph, Castle and now Merrison; Left, Right; Blue, Red; Bevan, Lobby, jobs; Supply, Demand; RAWP. And now a spoon named Vaughan. We sink deeper.

. . . Salmon, Joseph and now Merrison. As the years roll by, though one acquires a more historical perspective, it is still difficult to restrain one's anger with their almost total irrelevance to the job which the shopfloor worker in the NHS is trying to get on with. There is only one criterion on which they can be judged: have they or have they not made it easier for doctors and nurses (and many others) the better to look after patients? Do they preserve the integrity of the coin or do they crack it?

Bureaucracy cannot run health services

At no time in my experience has Nursing Management, for example, ever asked (even themselves, let alone out loud), 'Is Salmon working? Has it helped? Is recruitment better? Has the standard of nursing risen? Does the front line nurse in theatre, on the wards or in other departments feel better supported than before?' Attitudes in the NHS have become entrenched and view, say, Salmon as Revealed Truth which has been handed down from on high to be consolidated and perpetuated and not to be tampered with. This attitude is prevalent among Nurse Managers who are well placed to do the perpetuating. Do they, by and large, really speak for the front line nurse? Could they, even now, find a little humility and say, 'It is time for review: has it worked?'

Bureaucracy is inflexible and insensitive. A bureaucrat, most of us forget, is not an office worker (we need them), but an office ruler. What ruler readily relinquishes power? A bureaucratic system, rule by the office, is quite inappropriate for a service whose *raison d'etre* is to bring relief to ill and injured people. It is a system which does horrible things to people who enter it – nice people, well intentioned; but once inside they perpetuate and compound the disorder even as they assume they are doing a grand job.

VI

The Abuse of Man (and woman)- Power

Anne & Reuben Grüneberg

Dr Anne Grüneberg: A Consultant Anaesthetist at Harefield and Mount Vernon Hospitals. Honorary Secretary, Medical Women's Federation; member, General Medical Council; joint secretary, Hospital Consultants and Specialists Association; member, Central Ethical Committee of the BMA.

Dr. Reuben Grüneberg: Consultant Microbiologist, University College Hospital where he is Chairman of the Medical Committee and member of the Central Committee for hospital medical services. Chairman of the Area Medical Advisory Committee and of the North-East Thames Regional Pathology Advisory Committee. Council member, HCSA.

The NHS has lost Britain thousands of home-trained doctors who would have remained if British medicine had continued to develop freely. Dr Anne and Dr Reuben Grüneberg, one of our three man-and-wife joint authors, argue that the NHS misuses or under-uses the doctors that remain. They want bureaucratic "manpower planning" and nationally-fixed pay scales to be replaced by individual financial inducements to encourage recruitment to services and areas where bureaucracy has persistently failed to mobilise supply to meet demand. They point out that their views are personal and would be disowned by the organisations with which they are associated.

Introduction

The National Health Service is drifting aimlessly because people in positions of responsibility have forgotten its prime purpose. The NHS exists as a means of applying the skills of doctors, nurses and other professionals to meet the medical needs of patients. ("Health Service" is a misnomer – medical services cannot provide "health" but are concerned with prevention and treatment of disease).

When the aim of medical services is stated in this way, several sources of potential failure become evident:
    i. financial means may be lacking to achieve the aim;
    ii. available money may be badly spent;
    iii. there may be a lack of skilled manpower;
    iv. manpower may be badly aligned with the population it should serve;
    v. skilled manpower may be directed into irrelevant channels not directly related to the requirements of patients.

In our opinion all of these possible reasons for the difficulties of the medical services are, in varying degrees, relevant. In this essay, we consider aspects of the use of professional manpower.

The most important resource of medical services is its professional and skilled staff. The NHS is failing to use this resource appropriately. We propose a series of improvements which would be effective whatever changes in organisation may be introduced into British medical services in the next few years.

Hospital building neglected in the NHS

Medical services, however funded, cost a great deal of money. Most of it goes to the provision of hospital services. About 70 per cent of the total is paid in salaries. The NHS is the largest single employer in Europe. Its cost as a proportion of the Gross National Product is less than the expenditure on medical services in other industrialised countries.

It is arguable that it is inappropriate for much more money to be provided in the UK. If it were, better use ought to be made of it. Better use of money as well as of skilled manpower would require concentration of clinical activities in fewer, optimally-sized, hospitals.

It is generally recognised that hospitals in the UK should be mainly based on district general hospitals. It is also agreed that the hospitals should offer a full range of facilities and services. Units should either be purpose-built or appropriately modernised for their purpose, unlike the antiquated buildings full of health hazards in which we now struggle. This development would entail one District General Hospital of say 600–800 beds for each Health District serving a population of about 250,000 people, so reducing the number of general hospitals to just over 200. Concentration would reduce the number of beds by about a quarter, varying according to local circumstances. Specialist units and teaching hospitals would be additional.

For the past twenty years there has been reduction in the number of hospital beds and closure of units too small for a full range of services. There are signs that this process is accelerating.

The effect of having fewer, larger, more modern hospitals would be to facilitate more effective use of the existing professional workforce. This would improve the service to patients, raise staff morale and save money.

Before the NHS, there was a tradition of local communities taking pride in their hospitals and providing funds for them. Since then the hospital system has been starved of capital and buildings allowed to decay. What industry would expect to function with a capital expenditure of 3 per cent of its outgoings, as does the NHS? The few new hospitals, imposed on the local community and health professionals, have been grandiose concrete palaces unsuited to their function.

Unless money for capital projects is found, the hospital service will decay further. Scandals such as that following the highlighting of the dreadful state of the hospital buildings in the Normansfield Inquiry are bound to increase. Otherwise, implementation of draft Regional plans will lead to resistance and demoralising uncertainties, because changes will be seen as providing fewer facilities – not fewer and *better* ones.

Where can the capital money be found?
1. It could be transferred from current expenditure on running costs.
2. If the way medical treatment is funded in this country is changed, i.e. from taxation to insurance schemes, they could be designed to provide an initial injection of capital.
3. Reduction in the number of hospitals could lead to money being raised by the sale of surplus properties.
4. Local fund-raising could be encouraged by government matching pound for pound to help with building projects which satisfied simple nationally-agreed criteria. Once again, local communities would have a say in the hospital facilities available to them. The new District Health Authorities, acting on the advice of local health professionals and in consultation with local communities, could implement this policy.

Staffing of medical services: starving in the midst of plenty

The NHS has not succeeded in recruiting and retaining skilled professional staff. Although there has been a very large increase in the number of "health professionals" in the UK, as in other Western countries, since 1948 there nonetheless remains a serious shortage of key groups relative to demand. There are specialities in which recruitment is inadequate: in many areas, General Practitioners' lists of registered patients are too large for them to be provided with adequate attention; the pool of doctors has been supplemented by encouraging immigration; it is almost impossible to recruit trained Staff Nurses in London; there is a national shortage of Operating Theatre Nurses.

Under-supply is paralleled by under-use of skilled labour. Surgeons are unable to operate for lack of anaesthetists, theatre nurses or other staff. Trained nurses leave in droves because of poor pay and conditions of service, such as inflexibility of working hours. Medical emigration continues to seek better working conditions and pay overseas. Rising numbers of women doctors are not able to combine inflexible postgraduate education with part-time work. In the NHS, medical services are starving in the midst of plenty.

Two major forces create these defects. First, poor manpower planning, and, secondly, nationally-fixed salaries and conditions of service. Manpower planning in medicine, for example, has been totally unsatisfactory, producing vast swings from glut to famine in the supply of doctors as each Commission or Enquiry has recommended changes of policy. The same applies between medical specialities. Despite attempts to regulate the numbers entering each speciality (by the medical Establishment and the Health Departments acting in unholy alliance in the Central Manpower Committee), the number of doctors increases in the "over-subscribed" disciplines and does not expand in the specialities short of staff.

Meanwhile, the dead hand of fixed salary scales and terms of service precludes the correction of shortages, locally or nationally, by market forces. A false air of exactness arises in connection with manpower planning because numbers are applied to situations which cannot be accurately predicted. Rigid postgraduate educational requirements prevent flexible use of medical manpower when the demand for services shifts, for example, from treatment of tuberculosis to treatment of arthritis.

All attempts at speciality manpower planning or redistribution exercises should be abandoned. Central negotiations about health service salaries and conditions should only be concerned with basic terms of service and a minimum salary. This would restore the possibility of offering inducements for work in the under-subscribed specialities or areas. It would restore the possibility of offering flexibility to enable women doctors and nurses with family responsibilities to work part-time rather than not at all. It might help prevent medical emigration and make immigration less necessary.

Mis-use of manpower in irrelevant activities

What work should health professionals do? Doctors and nurses are selected and trained to look after the sick. Their efforts should not be diminished either by requiring all of them to spend a large part of their time in administrative duties or by separating off many of them as an administrative caste with largely non-clinical duties.

Every hour spent by a doctor in non-essential administration is a loss of one hour of skilled service. The amount of medical time taken by these administrative duties has increased, and is increasing. It should be diminished. The reasons for the increase are many, but are mostly concerned with the cumbersome administrative structure of the NHS with its many-tiered organisation. This loss of clinical time by involvement in administration is a potent source of poor medical and other professional morale. In spite of the time spent in this way by professionals in an *advisory* role, they are aware that all important *decisions* are taken elsewhere at Regional and Area Health Authority headquarters, and usually by people unaware of the individual or local realities.

"Community physicians"

There has recently arisen a new class of doctors called community physicians. They compute the "health care needs" (whatever that may mean) of the population, and are concerned with public health and preventive medicine. The last two of these functions are clearly necessary, but they should not require vast numbers of practitioners, nor a dominant position in the organisation of the Service. (There are more than three hundred of these doctors at the Department of Health alone, together with hundreds more in the Regional, Area and District organisations.) Although none undertakes significant care of patients they are listened to by the lay administration as though they were the only authorities on medical care. They are not accepted as such by clinical doctors in everyday touch with patients.

As a rule, the only doctors acceptable to their peers as administrators are those engaged in clinical activity who are elected by their colleagues to serve as their representatives for the time being. These elected professionals have their colleagues' support and trust and are in daily contact with clinical realities. Administrative medical advice can be more appropriately met by this means.

Administration should provide everything required by the doctors, nurses and others to serve their patient. This vital role of administration must be devolved to give the health professional confidence that decisions will be taken locally in full understanding of the realities. It would also free the professional staff from non-constructive time spent on administrative duties, to the considerable benefit of patients. What will also be necessary is a change in the attitude of health professionals, not least amongst doctors. Only when it becomes less respectable to sit pontificating about what others should do (as in writing this essay), than to do things for patients, will sanity return to the medical services.

Restrictive regulations reduce manpower availability

The problems of medical manpower utilisation have not all been created by governmentally-inspired bureaucracy. The professionals are also partly responsible.

The medical Royal Colleges (of Physicians, Surgeons, Obstetricians, and so on) have views about how and where postgraduate medical education should be conducted. The effect of the limitations imposed by them is to reduce the amount of direct medical service to patients. This is done by reducing the areas in which trainees can work and the tasks they are allowed to do, even under supervision. The only way a technique can be mastered is by doing it (under supervision) after having appreciated the principle and seen the practice.

There is a danger that these restrictions will be multiplied when the newly-reconstituted General Medical Council gets to grips with its new function of overseeing postgraduate education. Similarly, the requirements of the General Nursing Council and of the Council for Professions Supplementary to Medicine restrict the work done by trainees in nursing and laboratory techniques.

Women doctors wasted in hospitals – and now family doctoring

The cumulative effects of all these controls and restrictions can be illustrated by considering the difficulties faced by women doctors. A rising proportion of our medical students (currently approximately 38 per cent of medical school intake) is female. These expensively trained undergraduates expect, in due course, to be able to undertake responsible work commensurate with their skills. How does the NHS use them?

'It is the National Health Service which makes life difficult for women doctors', was the contention of Dr Jean Lawrie, a former honorary secretary of the Medical Womens' Federation. There is a contrast between family and hospital practice. In general practice most women doctors are working as principals alongside their male colleagues. This is because of the flexible way in which the provision of general practitioner services by independent contractors responding in some degree to market forces has evolved.

Vocational training regulations for general practice have now been passed by Parliament. This is the first time government has been given the opportunity of legislating on postgraduate education. One can imagine how difficult it will be to modify the structure of vocational training now it is enshrined in Act of Parliament.

It seems likely that, following the introduction of statutory requirements for postgraduate education in general practice, the employment of women doctors in general practice will change to resemble the under-use and abuse now prevalent in hospital specialities. Dr Berenice Beaumont's survey (*British Medical Journal 1978*) has shown that 91 per cent of women doctors under 60 are engaged in medical practice. (Note—Further aspects of the under-use of health professionals are discussed by Dr. Digby Anderson in Essay XIV—Ed.) It is when one considers what they are doing in their everyday work that the picture becomes depressing.

In England and Wales nearly 60 per cent of the women doctors employed in the NHS occupy non-training posts which do not carry complete responsibility for patients, although they are medically qualified and expected to take full responsibility. Many of them are working as clinical assistants or clinical medical officers, posts without security of tenure or career status. They are working as doctors but underusing their skills, to the disservice of patients.

Because many women doctors have responsibility for child care or the care of elderly relatives during the crucial period immediately after qualification, they should be able, if they are to use their skills fully, to:
1. complete postgraduate education, either full-time or part-time,
2. return to a medical career after a break, or
3. continue working though geographically tied.

The main reason why these options are not fully available is the rigid postgraduate "training" schemes and requirements. ("Training" in quotation marks because we consider "postgraduate education" more appropriate). The requirements are geared not to patient need but to the maintenance of the present pyramidal career structure in the hospital service, where for each consultant there are many junior doctors theoretically undergoing postgraduate "training". This state of affairs will continue unless:
1. a change in the way medical services are financed reduces the power of the Royal Colleges to veto flexible use of medical manpower, and provides incentives for consultants to undertake more patient care, instead of delegating much of it to junior doctors, or
2. the women doctors now qualifying obtain adequate public support for their contention that their potentialities should be taken into account. These should carry as much weight as the convenience of the medical Establishment and the wish of each Royal College to outdo the others in length of postgraduate "training".

In the past, this pattern of under-use of the skills of women doctors was perhaps of concern only to the individuals who had their early hopes of using their professional skills to the full blighted.

Since the Sex Discrimination Removal Act and the increase in annual intake into medical schools, the proportion and total numbers of women entering medical schools have been rising annually. There is thus blatant mis-use of an important national resource.

Summary

To enable medical, nursing and paramedical staff to do their best work it will be necessary to overhaul the medical services:

1. to concentrate general hospital activity into fewer, optimally-sized units;
2. to stop playing at manpower planning;
3. to permit financial inducements to be offered to aid recruiting to specialities or areas where supply of skilled staff falls short of demand;
4. to reduce the employment of health professionals in administration by:
   i. abolishing Area Health Authorities and Regional Health Authorities;
   ii. reducing "community medicine" to a realistic establishment and redeploying many of its practitioners to clinical duties;
   iii. relying on active clinical workers for professional advice on medical matters;
5. to reduce the ability of the Royal Colleges to interfere with clinical activity in the name of postgraduate medical education.

The policies would enable doctors, nurses and other professionals to do much more clinical work, to the benefit of patients all over the country.

VII
The Politically-Minded NHS is Endangering the Teaching Hospitals

George Bunton

Born 1920. M.Chir., FRCS. Educated Epsom College, Cambridge, and University College Hospital. Served in the RNVR. Senior Surgeon, Chairman, Medical Committee, and Member, Board of Trustees, University College Hospital. Chairman, South Camden District Management Team. Hon. Treasurer, University Hospitals Association (England & Wales). Member, Court of Examiners, Royal College of Surgeons.

So much for NHS general hospitals and their doctors. What of teaching hospitals – to which students come to learn medicine from all over the world? A senior surgeon at University College Hospital maintains that the NHS, obsessed with equality, is endangering the teaching hospitals. Successive governments, he maintains, have procrastinated long enough. Alternatives to the 'politically-orientated and politically-managed' NHS must be examined 'in deadly earnest'.

Introduction

If the provision of medical care in this country seems to be set upon a course of disaster, medical education is equally endangered. The long-term effects will be even worse. Not only are the University Hospitals and Schools responsible for producing some 3000 doctors a year; in addition, they provide training for most nurses and the para-medical services. Moreover, they engage in a larger amount of postgraduate education than the Postgraduate Hospitals themselves, important though these latter are in their specialities.

The economic plight of the country and central Treasury funding have prevented any effective increase in the money available for the NHS. Inflation steadily reduces the value of money that is available.

The proposals of the Resource Allocation Working Party (RAWP) were of serious concern to all University Hospitals because the principles were applied regionally in the distribution of resources. Although they might have been acceptable in theory, it is clear their validity and application in practice are highly questionable.

In 1948 Aneurin Bevan seemed to realise the value of University Hospitals and recognised it by preserving them with their Board of Governors. Subsequent events have hardly borne out the advantages which he and his advisers allegedly allowed to these institutions.

Conflict between long-term medical education and short-term treatment

Basically, the conflict lies between the long-term general needs of medical education and the short-term local needs of health care. These aims have come to be incompatible in the politically-orientated and politically managed NHS. Certainly some more far-sighted doctors realised this in 1948; 'You should not,' they said, 'bind yourself at the mercy of Governments that will come and go, whose policies and political complexion you cannot gauge, and whose handling of the health services will be dictated by political expediency'. 'The Ministry of Health,' said the late Sir Francis Walshe, 'is the politician's Didcot Junction on the way to Oxford'.

Cynical difference in treatment of general practice and hospitals

This political expediency has meant that the history of the NHS is littered with the debris of good intentions and bad decisions of successive ministers, whether Labour or Conservative. Increasingly in recent years the state of the country's economy has meant a comparative diminution in central government expenditure on health. It is however *politically* expedient to maintain general practice and community services at a standard which will satisfy the public, since the absence or deterioration of these services would be rapidly noticed by the public. The absence of adequate hospital resources (until last year) was less obvious. Therefore any shortage in general medical services is a matter of political sensitivity and they will always receive relatively high priority from funds dispensed with political motives. In contrast the University Hospitals have been studiously neglected by governments for reasons which were ill-founded.

The Department of Health has shied away from involvement with Universities and Medical Schools, since they are financed by the UGC through a different pocket of the

Treasury and have never wished to acknowledge that the involvement of Medical School Staff has taken over a substantial part of the commitments of the NHS. Equally the part played by the NHS consultants in the teaching of medical students is little recognised by the Department. The Universities themselves have become so poorly financed that the bulk of this work – and in many institutions half the teaching is done by non-academic NHS consultants and their juniors – is carried out with either minimal remuneration or, in some schools, no remuneration at all. Such a situation is regarded not only as ludicrous by authorities in other countries, but in some instances quite incredible.

Many doctors have long felt that University Hospitals were in some way protected from the full rigours of economic stringency. Partly because, before 1974, the Boards of Governors were answerable directly to the Department of Health and not to a Regional Authority, and partly because it was erroneously felt that they benefited somehow from both University funding and, in some cases, their own trust funds, there seemed little appreciation that a University Hospital must be extremely expensive.

To paraphrase the old Keith Prowse advertisement 'You want the best doctors – we have them'; but the best, like Rolls Royces, are costly. This feeling eventually led to the policy of re-deploying money and staff from University Hospitals to non-teaching hospitals, which it was argued were responsible for more of the local medical services for patients and should therefore receive an increase in funds and manpower. Yet where the future doctors were to come from to staff these hospitals and who would provide these monies was not very clear if the University Hospitals had to continue their role of training and teaching. Since a minority of doctors practise in University Hospitals, any policy of re-allocation will receive support from a majority of the profession. The public, conditioned by the Welfare State, can also be expected to support general medical services, with which it is mainly concerned. This view is frequently focussed by Community Health Councils, who, again for local political motives, are anxious to promote local medical services, so that a policy of devolving financial control further to local machinery is even less likely to benefit teaching interests. Therefore there is a climate in which politicians, the public and most doctors see a short-term advantage, either for personal or political motives, both central and local, which must result in seriously lowering the quality of future medical care in the training centres.

How to avoid another shortage of home-trained doctors?

Such policies will inevitably lead to a disastrous shortage of doctors of all kinds, with a marked fall in their quality. It is clear that such considerations were completely lacking in the 1974 re-organisation. Indeed the whole question of how teaching and the teaching hospitals should be dealt with, was left in the air; there was no one body responsible for their proper function.

The politicians and DHSS bureaucrats took refuge in saying that this was a matter for Regional and Area University liaison committees, which were found to be lacking both in responsibility and executive power. The Joint Consultant Committee consists overwhelmingly of members who hold no brief for the University Hospitals, though their original terms of reference included responsibility for the facilities available for teaching and research. The Royal Colleges, whilst laying down criteria for training and organising examinations to test the proficiency of students and doctors, equally had no say or responsibility for the organisation and running of University Hospitals.

Many believe that the BMA has some statutory responsibility in this sphere, not realising that, now a trades union, it exists only for the benefit of its members in negotiating terms and conditions of service, and as the only body through which government will negotiate with doctors. It has no say in running University Hospitals and training doctors. The newly-constituted General Medical Council, whilst it may lay down principles for the Medical curriculum in consultation with Universities, has no "authority" over teaching establishments. Indeed, only recently has the University Hospitals Association, consisting of the Deans of Medical Schools and Chairmen of Medical Committees of all the under- and post-graduate teaching hospitals in England and Wales, been able to form a responsible body to care for the fundamental interests of medicine and its teaching, through which government can seek advice and make its problems known in medical education.

What is a teaching hospital? The facile response that it is simply a hospital where medical students are taught does not stand up to scrutiny. Nevertheless this seems to be the answer that the Department of Health has accepted, apparently uncaring that the British teaching hospitals were slowly but surely losing identity and purpose. Indeed the Department has been so obsessed with the "service commitment" to the public that it appears to have completely lost sight not only of what a teaching hospital is, but also what it is for. Despite its concern with projections of medical manpower it would seem to think that more doctors will appear from some nebulous never-ending source.

Teaching hospitals are national and international

A teaching hospital can never be a district NHS hospital with students, administered by a Region or Area Authority and simply serving a local community or catchment area. It is welded to its medical school: the two are parts of one body and are indivisible. The hospital is tied to university commitments in a way that a district hospital cannot be, despite that students may attend district hospitals at intervals for part of their training and experience. A teaching hospital without its medical school ceases to exist as such; a medical school without its hospital is as surely decapitated as though guillotined. Teaching hospitals have not only a national but also an international role. The problems of administering such an institution are complex. Previously, the Boards of Governors were responsible for the hospitals with their Medical Committees; the School Councils with an Academic Board were their counterpart in the Medical School. Many members had a seat on both sides of the road, so to speak, and by the simple process of donning different hats, control and cross fertilisation of ideas flowed easily and freely between the two bodies.

Boards of Governors were assisted by a clerk or secretary to the Board. Seldom can any bodies have been served with more acumen, integrity and loyalty. To these men came dismissal or redundancy when the Boards were abolished; though a number were transferred to Regional or Area posts, many of the more senior chose retirement. Their direct experienced involvement with day-to-day running of the hospital was lost.

Teaching hospitals subjected to political influence and bureaucratic control

By the abolition of the Boards and their replacement by a District Management Team answerable to an Area Health Authority, answerable to a Regional Authority finally answerable to the Department of Health, the whole balanced structure between school and hospital was destroyed, particularly as medical representation on these bodies is very thin. The Area Authority is supposed to be analagous to a Board of Governors, but apart from three or four medical representatives, one of whom is the Dean of the medical school, and the others not necessarily representing the hospital, the remaining twenty or so members are local government officers and administrators whose knowledge or expertise in running any hospital, let alone a teaching institution is, to say the least, minimal. The 1974 Act, with its extra area tier, gave those doctors working in the hospitals and doing the teaching the feeling that their share in the control of the hospital was being totally eroded. They could now only see a vast inverted pyramid of bureaucracy leading up to the Elephant and Castle; a maze through which all communication was to filter up to some anonymous official and then equally laboriously, filter down again.

Even the simple process of appointing a single member of staff to a hospital involved the combined efforts of no less than seven separate committees.

Lord Smith of Marlowe, in commenting on these absurdities, once quoted a letter:
The NHS is the largest nationalised industry in Britain and the only one without a Chairman and Board of Directors. In place of a chairman it has had a dozen different ministers of health in the last thirty years, all of whom have had, in addition, an equally time consuming responsibility – i.e. that of Social Security.
A justifiable analogy might be to combine the Prudential Assurance Company with British Leyland and appoint a different man every other year to take on the responsibility of running the two, with the added proviso that no member of the workforce shall be paid more than three-quarters of the current rate for the equivalent job elsewhere.

With bureaucracy becoming overwhelmingly cumbersome, of increasing quantity and decreasing quality, many doctors feel they can no longer barter their medical skills for political dogma, nor entrust their ethos to a Department of poor ability.

As well set up a Ministry of Literature to tell Wordsworth how to write a sonnet.

It may seem strange that a group of institutions which have survived several hundred years of changing social structure and yet have steadily continued to produce the best of its kind in the medical world should in a few short years be considered outmoded and inefficient. Our teaching hospitals have been taken as models in all the Commonwealth systems, have been adopted in America. Such a spread of influence is hardly insignificant; indeed, the history of medicine over the last century is largely the history of the British teaching hospitals.

Their achievements have been reached by a tradition which has been formed by a succession of men inspired by great leadership and largely content to work for the cause of medicine rather than personal renown although the very nature of their work has made many of their names world famous. Some may not have been the best doctors in their day, but they were certainly among the outstanding teachers of medicine.

Destruction of irreplaceable values

The *Oxford Dictionary* defines education as 'forming habits, manners, mental and physical aptitudes – the culture or development of powers and the formation of character.' All doctors are the product of their teaching hospital but, whether Barts, Edinburgh or Newcastle, they carry its tradition and background for the rest of their lives. All owe a degree of loyalty and responsibility to the institution that gave them a scale of values and behaviour in medical adolescence.

It is this that a teaching hospital exists for; it is totally irreplaceable once it is lost. If the institution itself becomes debased the calibre of youg men and women prepared to work their way on to the staff will equally decline. There are already tell-tale signs in the number and quality of applicants for all grades of teaching hospital posts – academic and non-academic. A country may get not only the government but also the health service it deserves, but eventually it is medicine that suffers and consequently its patients. If the country denies those means and qualities of education required to produce good doctors, it must not be surprised or dismayed at the services it obtains. By antagonising young people who should be assuring posterity of its medical care and training, it is consuming its own seed corn.

A total failure of governments to appreciate this truth is at the root of the serious loss of morale among those whose business it is to teach medicine. It takes seven years for a student to emerge fully trained for the time of his acceptance, so that the ultimate effects will not show for some time. By then it will be too late, and it will probably not be possible to repair the damage for some fifteen to twenty years. Already university hospitals are having difficulty in maintaining standards. The prospect of having to increase the output of doctors without any further resources is viewed with mounting dismay. The problem is clear, if the country wants a continuing supply of good doctors it must be prepared to pay more taxes for them. If not, it must accept second or third best. If this is unacceptable to the public an alternative method of financing the hospitals must be urgently sought. The most obvious and efficient way of doing this is to introduce a market-orientated insurance system, based on tax-relief.

Change in financing essential

Despite the arguments increasingly voiced for economies – particularly in administration – these are quite impossible as the NHS is at present organised and financed.

First, such an enormous bureaucratic monopoly has been built up over the last thirty years that it has at last produced a system whose own needs now dominate those whom it should serve. Secondly, the underlying or concealed costs of such a vast machine consume some 20 per cent or more of the total cost of the NHS – certainly not the 6 per cent usually given in official answers. Thirdly, this system is controlled with political motives in mind and manipulated by the party which happens to be in power. Fourthly, the attitude of the trade unions engaged in health care precludes any attempt at a rational economic reorganisation of the NHS in its present pattern. Their interests have been clearly stated and, during the last few years, clearly demonstrated. They are emphatically not those of the patients.

As John and Sylvia Jewkes have pointed out: 'those obsessed with the case for equality will always be driven to seek out and destroy established centres of excellence. The British Teaching Hospitals with their outstanding reputation for research and advances in the higher levels of treatment have always been in danger since 1948'. This danger is now a real and immediate threat. It can only be described as social vandalism, abetted by the cardinal sin of procrastination, which is not only the thief of time but of talent and enlightenment as well. The days of procrastination are now numbered. The alternatives to the NHS must be examined in deadly earnest.

VIII
New Evidence on NHS Defects: A View from America

Cotton M. Lindsay

Born 1940. Educated University of Georgia, BBA 1962, Economics Major, University of Virginia, Ph.D 1968. Post-doctoral Fellow, London School of Economics, 1968–69. Asst. Prof. of Economics, UCLA, 1969–74. Associate Prof. of Economics, UCLA, 1969–74. Associate Prof. of Economics UCLA, 1974 to 1979. NATO Postdoctoral Fellowship in Science, 1968–69. National Fellow, Hoover Institution on War, Revolution and Peace, 1975–76. Distinguished Visiting Professor, Arizona State University, 1977. Professor of Economics, Emory University 1980. Numerous publications.

Then how does the outsider see the NHS? One of the two American economist contributors reviews the main findings of his researches in the NHS over two years. Resources have not been redistributed solely to areas of most "medical need"; on the contrary, shocking though it may sound, they have been channelled to areas where the political parties hoped to save or gain marginal seats. The NHS has not made the British healthier; the improvement in health since 1948 has been caused by forces that have improved health in other countries without a NHS, not least the USA and Canada. The NHS has not been more successful than other medical systems in meeting individual medical "needs", the NHS does not end rationing: its method of rationing by delaying treatment is not less arbitrary than rationing by price. The NHS does not improve medical care: it enlarges its quantity but lowers its quality. The NHS deals with appearances: it neglects the "invisible" but vital aspects of medical care.

Introduction

A study of the documents produced by Royal Commissions and various influential groups during the interwar years reveals two dissatisfactions with the British national health insurance of the period. First, it was believed that medical care was *distributed* badly by the national health insurance (NHI). British NHI did not cover the unemployed or even the families of workers, but the concern with the distribution results of NHI plainly extended beyond this uncovered population. Indeed, extension of NHI had broad support – even among the conservative bastions of professional medicine in the BMA and the Royal Colleges. Such an extension was rejected by those seeking a national health service on the grounds that insurance (even with universal coverage) failed to distribute care on the basis of medical "need", the only yardstick by which access to health care resources was judged morally acceptable.

Defective distribution and production

A second dissatisfaction concerned the organisation or the *production* of medical care. It was believed that medical technology had outgrown the existing institutions which were relied upon for the provision of nursing, hospital care and medical attention. The insurance system was centred on the general practitioner, while medical science was becoming increasingly focussed on the hospital. Modern medicine required teamwork, planning and co-ordination. It was believed that the existing diverse, local, voluntary, municipal and private suppliers were incapable of providing these advances in organisation. Only a national "service" with authority over all forms of health care could achieve efficient allocation of medical resources.

The champions of the NHS thus saw defects on both sides of the medical care market: supply and demand. The health care that was produced was not rationed among competing demanders appropriately, and its production was not organised efficiently. Government direction was sought for the first of these functions in order to divert care to regions and population groups considered underserved by the incomplete insurance system. Government planning and authority over the use of resources was sought in the name of the second – to improve the efficiency with which medical care was supplied.

An interesting irony presents itself here in the current political health debate in the United States. National Health *insurance* is advanced today in America for these very same reasons: unmet "needs" and organisational inefficiency. A system which was found *deficient* in these two central respects by the British is thus advanced as the *solution* to these same deficiencies in the United States! I here survey some results of a recent study: *National Health Issues: The British Experience* published in the USA (1980) in which I sought to shed light on the day-to-day achievements of the NHS in correcting these defects.

In this study I question the *validity* of familiar notions about markets, insurance and government organisation. Serious issue may be taken, for example, with the notion that "medical need" as a concept can be employed to make judgments about the efficient use of resources. An economist could also take issue with the argument that government can be shown to have inherent advantages over market institutions in even simple production.

Distribution under the NHS

Consider the question of access to care: Professors Cooper and Cuyler found in 1970 no tendency in the first two decades of NHS experience towards reallocation of health resources toward the regions which appeared to be under-served by the pre-NHS regime. Professor Rudolph Klein (and others) in the widely-cited Liverpool study in 1972 provided additional evidence that other factors besides "need" seem to be influential in allocating resources among patients.

Our 1978–1980 study took a different tack. We reasoned that, if the NHS was better serving the health "needs" of the population, its impact should be observed in the statistical "indicators" compiled to measure health internationally. We therefore examined a series of such statistics for evidence that the NHS had made the British healthier.

We sought to test the view, or claim, that adoption of the NHS in Britain made everyone healthier. Unfortunately, analysis of "health indicators", such as life expectancy is typically hampered by two statistical obstacles. International comparisons of these indicators, which might be made to reveal the supposed result, are clouded by the important influence of cultural, dietetic, genetic and economic factors which also influence the state of health under *all* systems. The incidence of heart disease, for example, varies widely from country to country for reasons which clearly have little to do with whether health care is organised by government or in the market. The influence of these factors can be excluded by restricting the comparisons to British experience before and after NHS adoption. This procedure, however, introduces a second problem. The new ("after") arrangements will be wrongly given credit for health improvement due to improving medical technology, not to government control. The introduction of the NHS had little to do, for example, with the eradication of poliomyelitis and tuberculosis. These diseases were brought under control in the United States *without* an NHS at the same time that they were controlled in Great Britain. Because of the timing of the introduction of the NHS, however, such before-and-after comparisons make it appear that state medicine substantially reduced the incidence of these diseases in Great Britain, a conclusion that cannot be drawn from the evidence.

Has the NHS improved British health?

We avoided these problems by devising a test which isolates the influence of the factor we wished to observe (changed *institutions* from market to government) for both these potential disturbances. This was done by observing the influence of the adoption of the NHS on *differences* in British and American health over time. As health technology is likely to reach the countries compared at roughly the same time, the effect of the introduction of polio vaccine, for example, will not be noticed in any difference in life expectancy between the countries. Cultural and other non-organisational factors will affect the amount of this difference, but their effect is likely to remain stable over time. By observing the behaviour of these *differences* over time, we are therefore able to identify changed *relative* positions between the countries examined, which may be attributed to the influence of the change from market to government. Thus, a marked improvement in life expectancy in Great Britain relative to the US after 1948 would suggest that adoption of the NHS had improved British health. On the other hand, no change in relative positions would indicate no identifiable effect of the change from the pre-war position to the NHS.

Our statistical tests for the influence of the NHS on health failed to refute the supposition that *the change in institutions (from voluntary/compulsory insurance to NHS) had no impact on British health*. Furthermore, a similar test between Canada, which has national health insurance, and the United States, which relies on privately purchased health insurance, found that the adoption of Canadian NHI also failed to improve measured health.

Medical "need" a red herring

Indeed, one is drawn to the conclusion that medical "need" is a red herring drawn across the path of the debate over the proper role for government in medicine. People who "need" medical care find it. They may pay for it in a market out of their own pocket or with the help of insurance. They may find it in the wards of municipal hospitals or in the voluntary ministrations of physicians in private practice. They may find it in government-insured clinics in Canada or NHS hospitals in the United Kingdom.

Institutions may affect the *way* is it delivered; whether in austere circumstances or in frilly packages. Institutions may determine whether someone gets all the care and attention he would like at the price charged. Evidence suggests however, that *institutions do not influence the satisfaction of peoples' "needs"*. It would seem, furthermore, that if people's basic "needs" for care are equally satisfied by various institutional arrangements, it would make sense to choose among those alternatives on the basis of *efficiency*, that is, by determining which produces the style of medical care that people want at lowest *cost* and gets it to the people that want it most.

Rationing by delay (NHS) more arbitrary than rationing by money

The second part of our analysis, therefore, consisted of assessing the performance of the NHS in organising the production and distribution of medical care. Getting rid of the market system and the profit motive in medicine makes political rhetoric. Designing a system to replace the valuable functions performed by these institutions is no easy task. It is not accomplished simply by the wave of a bureaucratic wand. A market rations medical care on the basis of the peoples' willingness to give up money to obtain it. This seems a totally unacceptable system to some, and reasonable to others. The architects of the NHS hoped to replace market rationing by price with a system which made medical "need" the criterion for access. In the event, however, they merely replaced one form of rationing with others which are at least as arbitrary.

Apart from cases of emergency requiring instant attention (which in real life are handled quite similarly under all health systems), we find that much hospital care under the NHS is rationed on the basis of *delay*. People *willing to wait longest* in order to move to the top of the list are eventually admitted. Those whose conditions will respond to self-treatment or outpatient treatment before their turn arrives (or, alternatively, find it uneconomic to wait and seek treatment outside the NHS) are denied access. Our statistical analysis of hospital waiting lists provided convincing evidence that rationing by delay is an important feature of the NHS.

Economic incentives in the NHS based only on measurable performance

Organisation of medical care production by government does not automatically ensure that the officials or others doing the organising are free of the influence of economic incentives. On the contrary, members of government organisations are as concerned with their economic positions as are their counterparts in business. They know the importance of the *appearance* of success in their jobs and the influence of their *perceived* performance on keeping their job and on their chances for professional advancement. Discovering how a government agency will perform, therefore, involves the discovery of how the *appearance* of success within such an organisation is achieved.

In our analysis, we studied government as an institution allocating resources where managers compete with one another in producing the "visible" aspects of medical care output which can be monitored by their superiors. But since much output of great potential value – such as choice – cannot be economically observed by higher officials, bureaucratic production presents scope for serious misallocation of resources. It gives rise to an aspect of NHS output that is, unfortunately, all too familiar in the outputs of other government agencies: *attention to quantity at the expense of quality.*

Analysis of real-life NHS operations provides much supporting evidence that this bias is present and important. That the NHS spends less per capita on health care than American medicine may reflect the relatively weak management incentives associated with government organisation more than any supposed gains in efficiency due to central planning. We observed in our study a distressing decline in the pay of doctors in Britain. It has resulted in the replacement of home-trained physicians (induced to emigrate by the low economic rewards in the NHS) by less well trained immigrant doctors. The NHS employs fewer personnel per available hospital bed, and has devoted far less to capital investment over the past thirty years. Although hospital beds are scarcer in the United Kingdom than America, patient stays in Britain are longer. This can only be rationalised by a system which puts management premium on lowering the *visible* cost per patient per day to the exclusion of more costly but higher-valued *invisible* uses of these resources. The cost of providing merely "hotel" services for patients awaiting surgery, or who have recovered, is certainly lower than the cost of treating patients requiring constant nursing or access to costly capital equipment. Hospitals anxious to give the *appearance* of cost effectiveness are therefore influenced to keep beds filled with patients whose demands on staff and equipment will be light.

Political influence in regional distribution of NHS funds

Internal management is not the only factor to impose its stamp on resource allocation by government. Government is first and foremost a political institution. The average citizen would probably be surprised if politics had no influence on most government spending. Analysis of NHS spending provides evidence that it is no exception. We analysed the spending of NHS funds between regions to determine whether they had been employed by the party in power to attempt to influence coming elections. A shrewd party leader would be expected to use the budget to "buy" votes by spending disproportionate amounts in marginal constituencies where results are expected to be close. The results of our statistical analysis confirm beyond any reasonable doubt that politics play a role in the budgetary decisions of the NHS.

In summary then, the NHS was adopted in response to real or alleged defects in the way that an insurance-based system distributed care and allocated health resources. Our analysis indicates, however, that the NHS operates with similar and perhaps more critical defects on both sides of the market. First, on the side of demand, though it has banished price, it has not banished the task of rationing. We find that the NHS system which performs this rationing is no less arbitrary than a price system. Secondly, on the side of supply, allocation of resources by government avoids the blinkered preoccupation with profit, but profit considerations can produce beneficial results in allocating resources. Furthermore, when government does the allocating instead of firms, we replace profit by politics in the centre of the decision calculus. The analysis of such results for general welfare is far from complete in the current state of economics. But it seems doubtful whether even the occasional correspondence between self-seeking behaviour and social good observed in a market can be expected of government control and financing.

IX
The Mis-Use of Medicines

W. Duncan Reekie and Ruth J. M. Reekie

Duncan Reekie: *Reader in Business Economics, University of Edinburgh. Co-author of "Profits, Politics and Drugs". Has written extensively in the professional journals on the economics of the pharmaceutical industry. 1970–73, on the industry's Economic Development Committee (or "little Neddy"). Has taught in the Universities of Strathclyde, Toronto, the Witwatersrand, Johannesburg and Pace, New York.*
Ruth Reekie: *MB, ChB, General Practitioner in Fife.*

Then is the NHS better at ensuring access to medicines? Dr. Duncan Reekie, an economist at the University of Edinburgh, and his wife, Dr Ruth Reekie, a family doctor in Fife, reply that the NHS has prevented the patient from benefitting from technological advances and made costs higher thay they could be. The low charges for expensive medicines encourages over-use of drugs prescription and the under-use of over-the-counter "home medicines". Moreover, surgeries are unnecessarily crowded, the shortage of doctors is made all the more harmful to patients, the chronic and seriously sick are further burdened, and the poor remain poor. Poverty should be dealt with differently from ill-health: low incomes require separate treatment; medicines should carry their full price.

Introduction

The cost of drugs is low. The benefits from pharmaceuticals conversely are enormous. The benefits in turn lower the total cost of medical care in either state or market systems. The argument of this essay is that we cannot reap the full economies which drugs potentially provide unless they are supplied by a free market mechanism.

The cost of drugs

In 1979 the average cost of a prescription to the NHS was £2.44 (including the dispensing fee). This is absolutely low. It is also low in relative time. At £972m in total the nation's drug bill has remained constant at around 8–10 per cent of the total cost of the NHS for three decades. And this has occurred despite the fact that the number of prescriptions written has increased by about 75 per cent from 215 to 375 million per annum.

The benefits from drugs

The results are the obvious benefits of better health and all that implies. TB mortality has fallen away dramatically since the introduction of streptomycin, PAS and isoniazid. During the first four years of the NHS, shortage of TB beds was considered a major defect of the system. The Ministry of Health had top priority plans for building new sanatoria. Meanwhile the pharmaceutical industry discovered, tested, developed, mass-produced and marketed anti-TB drugs which swept the whole scourge of TB away. In 1953 there was still a big shortage of beds. By 1955 the shortage had gone, and tuberculosis beds were closed in ever-increasing numbers.

The death rate among children has declined continuously since the mid-nineteenth century. Better sanitation and improved social and economic conditions have been the contributory factors. In the late 1930s, however, the rate of improvement in mortality rates accelerated rapidly. Coincidental with the change was the introduction of new medicines and vaccines capable of preventing or curing many previously fatal diseases. Had the 1900–1935 downward trend continued (and not accelerated) 7500 more children would have died in 1968, for example, than otherwise. At least half of these "saved lives" were due to the near-eradication of deaths from pneumonia, TB, diphtheria, measles and whooping cough: and all thanks to the products of the competitive pharmaceutical industry, not to the NHS.

How drugs lower the cost of medical care

The discovery of the first of the tranquilisers in 1952 and of the anti-depressants in 1960 led to the start of psycho-pharmacology. Psychotherapeutic drugs were a major cause in 1956 of the first ever annual decrease in the number of occupied hospital beds due to mental illness. From 151,000 in-patients in 1956 the number of mentally-ill hospital patients fell to 125,000 in 1966 and to 80,000 by 1977.

This advance was parallelled in other diseases. New drug products enabled the GP to assume functions previously undertaken by the hospital consultant. It has been said that 'today the practitioner in the gloomiest slum practice can treat pneumonia more effectively than the most eminent specialist could before the War'. If we bear in mind the relative money prices of average cost of a prescription (£2.44), and the NHS hospital cost per in-patient week (£310 in 1979), the degree to which pharmaceutical research, development and innovation has resulted in medical care economies is dramatically highlighted.

Although this pharmaceutical development has resulted in increased usage of the GP services of the NHS, the average cost to the NHS of a visit to a GP (including drugs and the GP's income and practice expenses) is only around 3.5 per cent of that of an in-patient week and 2.0 per cent of that of an in-patient's full treatment period.

This, of course, in a "socialist" medical system brings about corresponding dis-benefits: misuse of the GPs' consultation time and consequent dangers of over-prescribing. A "free" consultation and prescription (or a prescription with a nominal charge considerably below costs) results in the demand for these services exceeding their supply. Patients with trivial complaints fill GPs' waiting rooms; in self-defence the GP rations his services. Even doctors must sleep. There are only 24 hours in a day, and only 26,000 GPs in the country. Since he cannot ration by price, the GP resorts to rationing by time to balance demand with his available time and expertise. He provides patients with an average consultation of 5 minutes, a *quarter* of the time his therapeutics professor in medical school emphasised (20 minutes) as the optimum length of patient examination. And to help "clear his surgery" he writes prescriptions which may be unnecessary or, given the pressure of events on his judgment and skills, even harmful.

Thus although drugs lower the costs of medical care universally, they do so less effectively under a state system. A market system would more effectively remove the dis-benefits resulting from the overcrowding of GP surgeries.

Charging an economical price for medicines: advantages and disadvantages

Prices are signals. They pass messages to people that goods or services are not endlessly available. To charge patients an average price to cover costs per prescription would illustrate this more effectively than the current zero price for exempted cases and 70p per item for others which covers only one-twentieth or so of costs. Even £1 per prescription would cover around a third of costs.

Charging for medical care as a whole will have to come sooner or later. Charging for pharmaceuticals may be the simplest place to start since the price of a script is low and the retailing mechanism exists in the form of pharmacy outlets. It would not require an abrupt change in national habits. Even a low price paid to the family doctor would encourage patients to consider whether or not their visit to the doctor was essential relative to other claims on their time. The charge would reduce the number of calls made on the GP's time, and so permit him to improve the quality of his examination and treatment. It would also decrease the abuse of over-prescribing and so lower the nation's drug bill as a whole.

The obvious drawback of charging is that some patients who have a genuine requirement to visit a doctor may forego essential medical care. This argument can be neatly pushed on one side, however. The problem we are discussing is the efficient allocation of health care resources, not that of poverty. The advantages of charging could be retained and the disadvantages of poverty overcome by subsidising people, not drugs, by some form of reverse income tax, voucher scheme, or by compulsory, but subsidised private health insurance.

Without prescription: beneficial home medicines

Even patients with minor complaints who are discouraged from visiting their GP by drug charges would not disappear from the medical care market. The home medicine industry provides drugs available for sale to the general public without prescription. It is no accident that Britain, with its "free" NHS, has the smallest home medicine industry in the developed world. In 1977 it accounted for 0.5 per cent of total retail sales while in Germany, Australia and the USA the corresponding figures were 1.5 per cent, 3.2 per cent and 1.9 per cent.

Self-medication is relatively unimportant in Britain. Yet the Price Commission in its review of the industry in 1978 said 'the availability of such medicines . . . reduces the calls on doctors and assists them in deploying their skills to the best advantage. The NHS would be quite unable to deal with the extra demand which would be unleashed in the absence of medicines for sale over the counter . . .'.

The responsible consumer

Moreover studies show that the general type of complaints treated by the individual include worry, nervousness, headaches, coughs, colds and sore throats, back aches and "tummy troubles" and the like. These are exactly the ailments doctors have stated are most suitable for self-medication.

In short, the home medicine industry is treated responsibly by consumers and is not used as an alternative for valid medical consultations. Self-treatment shifts the responsibility away from the NHS onto individuals themselves. It is a part of health care which could be expanded as the traditional principles of self-reliance and self-care in health matters are revitalised. Doctors, pharmacists and the industry's advertising all have an educative role to play in encouraging and ensuring the proper use of home medicines. As *Which?* has said 'Self-medication is part of the routine of living'.

Yet government action so far has removed both these actual and potential benefits and further raised the costs of health care.

Increasing the pressure on the NHS by further regulation

Since the passing of the Medicines Act in 1968, exit from the industry has been widespread. Manufacturers have been subject to the granting of licences. As the 1978 Price Commision Report stated, 'the standards required to satisfy the licensing authorities have led some companies discontinuing a variety of products and even to abandon manufacture altogether'. In other words, costs have been raised and the wealthier consumer who can, and is prepared to, buy from the higher cost manufacturer is duly protected. The producer with the higher costs (because of advertising or inefficiency) is in turn protected from the lower-cost firm which previously sold to more price-sensitive consumers. Some of these consumers are thus driven back to the "free of charge" GP, imposing further on his time and resources.

Similarly, from 1978, promotion of home medicines for certain diseases has been banned, with adverse consequences for consumer knowledge and so choice of treatment. In addition sales of some medicines have been banned unless they pass through a retail pharmacy; so have analgesic packs containing over 25 tablets. The Price Commission noted that such changes are 'significantly eroding price differentials'. That is, they remove the manufacturing economies which many smaller firms possess because of low advertising budgets but localised and intensive, low-cost distribution networks. They can no longer be set against the marketing and innovation advantages of larger companies that typically sell at a higher price and already supply the non-pharmacist in small packs.

Conclusions

1. Pharmaceuticals, both prescription or over the counter, are inexpensive. They have provided rapidly rising medical benefits over the last three decades with no increase in cost. Conversely the total cost of medical care has been reduced as drugs are both cheaper and more effective than many alternative remedies.
2. But the economies which society could reap from this development have not been fully realised in the NHS.
3. Medical costs are higher than they need be. Doctors' surgeries are overcrowded.
4. Prescriptions may be written for the wrong reasons. The home medicine industry, which could, in principle, remove some of the pressure on the NHS is discouraged, and its prices are made higher than they otherwise would be.
5. The problems of poverty, doctor shortage and those of chronic and serious illness are thus accentuated.
6. Decontrol of the over-the-counter market and the introduction of full economic pricing for prescription medicines would go far to remove these deficiencies.
7. Poverty should be tackled as a problem in its own right, not as an issue involving the price of only one of society's myriad of goods and services.

X
A Better Way to Pay
for Dental Services

David Smith

Professor of Dental Radiology at London University. Teaches at King's College Dental Hospital School. Four years on Southwark Borough Council. A member of the Greater London Council and Leader of the Opposition on the Inner London Education Authority. Member, South East Thames Regional Health Authority.

So much for family doctor and hospital services. Dentistry has suffered from similar strains in coping with scarce resources that have to be rationed arbitrarily because they have no price or a price below their cost. Professor David Smith reveals in dentistry the same NHS pre-occupation with quantity and the relative neglect of quality revealed by Professor Lindsay in family doctoring and hospital services. Even more in dentistry than in family doctoring, patients, at first in the affluent South East and spreading gradually to the industrial North, are rejecting the NHS because they are ready and able to pay for better services.

Introduction

When the NHS was instituted in 1948, dentistry was seen as an integral part of it. But the extent of the pent-up demand for dental treatment had not been appreciated. The newly created general dental services were immediately subjected to very considerable stress. More fundamentally, not only had the demand for dental treatment been underestimated, but the financial implications of a "free" (although for only a short initial period) dental health service had not been foreseen.

Some of these financial repercussions were the result of the method by which dentists are paid. Since the inception of the NHS, general dental practitioners have been paid by item of service. It very soon became apparent that, because so much work was available, they were able to earn very much more than had originally been anticipated. Predictably, the Government's response was to cut back on the scale of fees and so reduce the incomes of the NHS dental surgeons.

Drawback of target income from fee for services: lower quality

It was not long before it was realised that an item-of-service method of payment had drawbacks when linked to a target net income. It was, in effect, a productivity scheme with a built-in regulator which ensured that *increased* work and output was followed by a relative *reduction* in the amount of fees. The results of the profession's negotiations with government had set dentists on to a treadmill which could only go faster. The fees that dentists received for each item of service became smaller and smaller relative to those paid for similar work in other countries. This ill-designed system of payment has undoubtedly had the unfortunate result that the temptation to maximise income by producing mediocre work has become very real.

It was not only in dentistry that NHS costs were larger than anticipated. The Treasury soon began to express alarm about the developing trends. Eventually it led to the Guillebaud Committee in 1955 to report on the cost and organisation of the NHS. But even before this event a Labour Government had in 1951, to introduce charges for some types of dental treatment and for prescriptions. These branches of the NHS were chosen, I suspect, because it was administratively simple to collect the money by these means.

Misuse and use of charging

Over the years, once the principle of charging had been accepted, each successive financial crisis saw the Ministry, now the Department, succumbing to Treasury pressures and raising the charges for dental treatment in order to reduce the tax contributions. These charges in some instances, as for dentures, became a very significant part of the whole cost of treatment. Although expensive to the patient, the fees paid to the dentist in many cases only barely covered the cost of any laboratory work required, so that there is little or no recompense to the dentist for his work. The inevitable happened: some dentists became reluctant to do certain kinds of dentistry, especially those requiring laboratory work. Patients became aggrieved because these were the items for which they had to pay (by customary low NHS standards) substantial amounts.

The main economic argument for charging for a service rather than providing it through taxation is that taxes can be reduced, leaving people with more money to spend, and so extending personal choice. This economic philosophy has to apply to a substantial proportion of income for it to work. The total cost of dentistry is very small compared to spending on the rest of the NHS. So, although charges are levied for dentistry, there is no corresponding reduction in taxation. Dentistry is thus effectively being given the worst of both worlds.

There is a strong case for shifting the burden of payment for the NHS from direct taxation to patient charges in actuarily designed private insurance, with appropriate safeguards to ensure that treatment is possible within the high-cost, high-technology specialities, and that provision is made for people suffering from serious chronic illness or disablement. But the decision to charge for dental services and not for other aspects of medical care can be challenged on clinical as well as economic grounds.

There is no justification for patients paying for treatment for an abscess at the root of a tooth, but not if it is anywhere else in the body! Dentistry must be seen as an integral part of the total health care of the patient. The financial arrangements for dentistry must not conflict with those for medicine. The time has come for new thinking: a substantial portion of the funding should come from charges rather than taxation.

Payment for preventive dental treatment

The other continuing mistake that has been made by NHS policy-makers is their refusal to countenance proper payment for preventive dental measures. Since the inception of the NHS, preventive techniques, which include instruction in oral hygiene and dietary advice, have made significant strides. Much dental disease today would not occur if dentists were encouraged to practise preventive dentistry by being paid for it. Certainly the NHS has seriously distorted the progress of dentistry in Great Britain.

Better health without the Health Service

The success of the NHS is all too often assessed by comparing the undoubted progress contrasted with the state of affairs that existed before 1948. (Professor Lindsay examined the statistical evidence in Essay VIII—Ed.) A more realistic assessment would be to compare the state of the nation's health today against what it *might* have been had there been no NHS.

During the last thirty years there has been a dramatic increase in the standard of living in the United Kingdom. There can be little doubt that there would have been a marked increase in the standard of medical care whatever the method of organising it. What should be asked is whether, with appropriate (perhaps statutory) insurance schemes, the private sector would now be providing better health services than that provided by the NHS. In dentistry, I suspect the answer to that question might be *Yes*.

XI
Over-Centralisation and its Uniformity Unsuitable for Medical Care

Roger Eddison

Has undertaken research studies for planning in large organisations, particularly transport and health services, in many countries. Past President of the Operational Research Society. Visiting Professor in Operational Research at the University of Sussex, 1968–1974.

Then what about management? Are health services perhaps organised better in a centralised structure like the NHS? Professor Lindsay in Essay VIII produced evidence to the contrary. Here Roger Eddison, a specialist in the study of large-scale organisation, is not at all sure they have been, or can be. Health services, he argues, must be decentralised *so that the people on the spot, who* know *more than planners at the centre take the decisions. Give local people power to exercise the desired controls as* they *think best. Above all, let patients choose the services they want – with advice and guidance from people they trust. The question is whether all this decentralisation is possible – probably – in the NHS where the money is controlled at the centre. It is tackled in other essays.*

Introduction

The words "centralised" and "decentralised" when applied to an organisation refer essentially to the decision-making process within it. We are concerned with organisations of people consisting of separate parts each of which may have its own interests and objectives to satisfy. The parts work together as an integrated system in order to obtain advantages, for example sharing specialised effort, so that the benefit of the whole will be larger than the sum of the benefits of each part separately. This process inevitably requires some sacrifice in freedom of choice by the separate parts, which may have to adjust their objectives so that they become consistent with one another. Thus the smooth working of an organisation entails the balancing of interests by a process of give and take.

NHS purpose to serve the individual

The NHS is such a system. It is about people; the basic unit is the individual with his own various ideas about the kind of service he thinks would be best for him; without that, the NHS would have no purpose. But it is also made up of people working as units of varying size and complexity – from individual doctors, nurses, pharmacists and many others, through local health centres or community hospitals to large general or specialist hospitals, and to the NHS as a centralised entity.

The problem in structuring the decision-making processes for such an organisation is how to maintain a balance between the interests and ensure that all activities decided upon are consistent with the objectives of the entity and of its parts. It may seem obvious that, if the various objectives in the system are to be satisfied by consistent decisions, this result may best be achieved by central, "authoritative", decision-making. So, as organisations become larger and more complex, they will tend to be *seen* as requiring a centralised structure together with the communications and skilled administrative service that it requires. The eminent Soviet management scientist Gvishiani, no doubt influenced by arrangements in the East, observes this as a general trend in the West. He sees the formalisation of management processes giving more power to specialist administrators, with a consequent movement towards the centre of the boundary between planning and performance. Just when the systematic advantages of more centralised structures are becoming more beguiling, computer technology is making available the means of providing them.

Centralisation tends to uniformity

The trouble with centralisation is that uniformity is very difficult to avoid. The structure tends to become expensive and to create its own internal demands whose satisfaction receives priority over freedom of choice in the performance of personal services. The variety of response is reduced, and the speed of response may be slow. In short, it provides what Schumacher called the orderliness of order but at the expense of the disorderliness of freedom. His solution was not "either-or" – centralisation or decentralisation – but both at once. The mixture will vary with different kinds of decision.

In industrial organisations the tendency of internal requirements to take charge can be seen for example, in the restriction of variety of product in order to obtain the managerial and production advantages of long production runs: the problem of the so-called production-orientated company. It was Henry Ford who was reputed to have said 'People can have cars any colour they like – so long as it is black'. There is of course a perfectly valid argument for standardisation. In a commercial setting the restriction of choice for the consumer can be treated as a simple matter of economics, measured and balanced against the lower prices made possibly by production economies.

In health services, on the other hand, the consumer's individual requirement may be absolute. Furthermore, it is a short step from suiting the convenience of the system to suiting the convenience of the people working the system; then we have bureaucracy and dirigism. In the NHS this kind of failure to take account of the consumer's wishes and convenience can be found in the appointment system which calls all patients in at the same time to avoid keeping any medical staff waiting ever: in the blood tests that can only be taken on Sunday ready for batch processing on Monday: in the X-ray that cannot be issued until seen by the radiologist who happens not to be there.

Size *v.* service

But the objection goes much deeper than that. Consider planning decisions on the broad strategy of the NHS – what to invest, where, and when. They are to do with the effect of such actions on the efficient functioning of the system to provide the desired results. The advantages of centralisation must, if anywhere, be seen at their best in planning. An interesting example is provided by the task of deciding hospital size. A decade ago it was fashionable to say that very large hospitals were most efficient, and some monsters were indeed approved for building. The argument for larger size was put in a committee report in 1969 on the functions of the District General Hospital published by the Central Health Services Council. It recommended that for planning purposes the maximum size for any hospital in an urban area – then taken to be 600–800 beds – should be doubled (or more precisely, that the size of population served by a single hospital should be doubled). This conclusion appeared to be based on one single argument – that each speciality in a hospital should support at least two consultants (for convenience and effectiveness of their work) and that the population to two consultants was less than 150,000 for only two specialities – general medicine and general surgery; so the population served by each hospital should be increased up to 300,000.

There are of course economies of scale and other advantages (of which consultants per speciality is only one) arising from large size in hospitals as well as in other enterprises; but there are also disadvantages. Some years after the 1969 report a research study was set up which took into account the effect of size on many factors including not only the *internal* administration and working efficiency but also such things as the building schedule and accessibility for staff, *patients* and *visitors*. The outcome was effectively to *reverse* the committee's recommendations!

That is an example of how NHS centralisation can easily fall into the trap of making a decision on a single, most obvious, factor. It also shows how, on the other hand, centralisation can reach decisions based upon a comprehensive analysis of a whole variety of relevant factors and upon observation of day-to-day behaviour in different circumstances. But a word of warning: to achieve the more complex purpose calls for a deliberate and substantial effort; and the example quoted is a relatively simple one. Consider how much more difficult it is to take adequate account of the huge variety of factors and effects involved in the conflict – or rather range of conflicts – encompassed in the phrase "balance of care", which may refer to prevention *v.* cure: or to services "in the community" as opposed to in-patient treatment: or to services for chronically ill patients as opposed to more glamorous acute work such as heart transplants.

The essential is variety

Variety is the nub of the matter. Patients suffer from a variety of complaints calling for a variety of treatments which may be presented to them and applied in a variety of forms. The task is to match the variety provided to the variety demanded, and furthermore to ensure that the matching can be made efficiently and quickly on the spot. This task can best be solved in decisions made when doctor meets patient. But it may be frustrated by the absence of the right resources, in which event the demand must be moderated to match the supply. The absence of the right resources may arise because of wrong planning decisions taken long beforehand; or it may be because of an inevitable element of rationing due to the economic impossibility of providing unlimited resources to meet every variety of demand.

Variety is important also in another slightly different contest. Medical services are at a stage of rapid evolution with fast-developing new technologies. Biological evolution relies upon the concept of survival of the fittest. If we accept the analogy, the evolution of an organisation or service must depend upon the testing of different ideas by trying them out in practice and by observing behaviour in each case, so that the best can be built upon.

Associated with limitation of resources is a need for control. In a public service especially, control has an important element of monitoring to ensure that public money is being spent properly. But the control wanted here is something much more subtle: it must be designed to ensure that the resources provided are used in the most effective way to match the demand as it arises. The theory of control in large organisations is complex. *The controls must have as much variety as the system they are controlling.* That variety is manifested and can have its most direct effect at the point where demand meets supply. Advantage should be taken of the self-organising possibilities of control at this point. Attempts to maintain control from the centre in a system such as the NHS (which requires high variety) become cumbersome and slow, and lead inevitably to further reduction in variety of choice. This is a cause of the uniformity that is one of the usual attributes of highly centralised decision making.

Decision-makers must know costs

To have the best chance of good co-operation between planning and execution and of efficient and unobtrusive control, decisions are best made by the person responsible for the result of the decision, which often means someone far from the centre. Nobody can make good decisions in the absence of information, especially on costs. This is often one of the reasons advanced in favour of a highly centralised system, on the grounds that only the spider at the centre of the web can know everything that is going on. But information can flow down as well as up to the centre. Modern information systems can be used to provide the executive at the periphery with information at his elbow to help him making decisions. In commercial practice this can be seen in the principle of making operating units into profit centres. But more than the physical means of spreading information is required. There must also be the *will* to share it; but secretiveness is the hallmark of the bureaucrat, especially of the bureaucrat who is unsure of himself.

All these arguments suggest that benefits will come from the highest possible degree of decentralisation in health services. Let the people who know, who have to perform the day-to-day services, make the decisions. Trust local communities by extending controls to them so that each can make decisions as it thinks best. Give patients the chance to choose the types of service they prefer. Keep decisions and controls at the centre only when that is the right place for them. More patients will then get more of what they want; staff will get more satisfaction from being able to do the job they know needs doing; and the country will get better value for money.

XII
The Hidden Costs

Francis Pigott

Born 1933. Trained at St Bartholomew's Hospital. Served in the RAF Medical Service. 7 years experience as a general practitioner, 7 years as an anaethetist. Spent four years in Canada. Now working for the British Medical Association. Medico political experience as a representative of junior hospital doctors and as a fee negotiator.

Since long before it began, advocates of the NHS claimed that as a centralised system it would cut out duplication, organise doctors and equipment efficiently, and not least cut down the costs of administering health services. Francis Pigott rejects this claim. He argues that the NHS has higher costs than shown in official statistics because it "hides" most of them by various devices. It shifts some costs to industry, to patients (and their families or friends), to taxpayers, and to our children in the future. Industry has to record tax and national insurance payments. Patients have to wait for consultations and then for treatment – and lose earning capacity (or time). They (and their visitors) may have to travel long distances. Taxpayers have to pay for temporary treatment, for unnecessarily expensive long-term treatment because patients are older and, for training doctors "driven out by the NHS". And our children (and grandchildren) will bear the costs of renewing hospitals and equipment run down by the NHS.

Introduction

Throughout its life the NHS has had its critics; it has also had many more defenders. After thirty years of intermittent warfare the defence lines are static and rigid, although the strategic emphasis has shifted.

The two major forts are: 'The NHS is the envy of the world' and: 'It is very cheap and good value for money'. During the last decade the first fort had become more or less swamped by a growing realisation that whilst we have had in *some* respects a *fairly* good health service, most other advanced countries have caught up with us or surpassed us. The other fort is now the key defensive point, flanked by newly erected works, such as 'We can do no more until the economy improves' and 'NHS administrative costs are low'.

In the United Kingdom less is spent on health care than in many similarly wealthy countries. One faction uses this statistic to prove that we ought to spend more; another to prove we are getting marvellous value for money. In the ensuing conflict we lose sight of the truth that we do not know the total costs of the NHS (or of any other health service).

Ignorance of NHS capital costs

Many recognisable indirect costs are not measured, even though the NHS has always had both compelling reasons to externalise or "export" them and an unrestricted ability to do so. There is a fairly general consensus that insufficient money has been spent on new hospitals, clinics and equipment. In many other countries most medical buildings have been replaced since the Second World War, and they will continue to be renewed or replaced at regular intervals. As the NHS has never valued its buildings and equipment and does not keep proper capital accounts, there is no way of computing the capital deficit accumulated already. Neither is there any way of keeping track of how it is going. A major part of the true cost of keeping the NHS going has been concealed so effectively that we cannot know what it is even if we wanted to know. In reality we are happy to let that cost be met by a future generation.

There has been a tendency to close smaller "uneconomic" hospitals and clinics and to concentrate services in fewer larger units. Although some studies have been done on the relative direct costs of small and large *hospitals*, there is no evidence that a systematic and complete review of the relative costs of each *service* provided has ever been undertaken. In the late 1960s a BMA panel considering financing of health services obtained information that indicated a unit cost increase of about 30 per cent in new hospitals built since the Second World War. Perhaps this early experience discouraged further research because the results would have embarrassed the supporters of the big hospital.

Exported/transferred costs

Closing local small facilities may result in some saving of money for government, but usually it throws a considerable financial burden on others. Patients have to travel further, spend more time travelling and often experience longer delays and waits when they eventually reach their destination. Patients' visitors experience similar difficulties and staff may find themselves redundant or spending longer travelling and having to pay more to get to work. Part of the increased cost is paid by individuals, some by employers and some by government – but out of another pocket. Although recently there has been some recognition of social costs, there is no requirement for the authorities to compute the external financial costs accurately and to show there is likely to be a real saving before they close an "uneconomic" unit.

Failure to provide adequate services or delayed access to treatment may cause large expenses for patients, their families or the State. There is good reason to believe that many of the tragic cases of children damaged at birth could be prevented. The total cost of this neglect is difficult to count, as much is borne by families, and we do not make adequate efforts to look after and educate these children. Many people become crippled by arthritis of the hip. A cure is available for most of them – replacement of the hip joint. For the majority who cannot afford private surgery there is a long wait for the operation. During the wait the family and social services have to spend a lot of money. There may be a further economic loss due to diminished earning capacity. The operation costs just as much when it is done eventually: indeed there may be increased direct costs because the patient is older and weaker, causing prolonged hospitalisation and rehabilitation. All the extra costs generated by delay is money wasted.

Delay raises costs

Delay in providing treatment for non-urgent conditions results in an incidence of avoidable complications such as strangulated hernias or bleeding from peptic ulcers which not only cause unnecessary suffering and even death, but also result in increased direct treatment costs.

One of the commonest complaints made by patients is that they do not have time to talk to the doctor. This leads to delay in diagnosis and treatment, unnecessary repeat visits to the doctor or hospital, over-investigation and unnecessary treatment with drugs. The associated unnecessary costs would be difficult to assess. The cost resulting from prolonged incapacity is even more difficult to measure, but may be even higher.

I have concentrated on the purely financial aspects of the argument because we have been encouraged to believe that running health services on the cheap makes good sense. At the same time we have been deceived because there has never been an attempt to measure the whole cost of such a policy.

The hidden cost of lost doctors

Even if it is possible eventually to justify underprovision on purely financial grounds, other indirect costs must be brought into the account. Since 1948 more than 10,000 British doctors have emigrated. Although some doctors would emigrate anyway, many have been driven out of the country by the NHS. In 1949 the decision to restrict the increase in numbers of hospital consultants resulted in many doctors having their training hampered and their careers blighted. Canada was one of the beneficiaries, and doctors with higher qualifications and impeccable references arrived to start practices. Initially there was a natural suspicion that they must have blotted their copy books and been forced to flee the country. On the contrary, they were among our best and most industrious graduates who would not tolerate the poor working conditions and rewards offered by the NHS. We have lost a whole cadre of hardworking clinicians with high standards who would have provided good care, maintained standards, and been available to train succeeding generations of doctors.

Official bodies have attempted to minimise the perception of this loss by referring to balances of numbers coming to this country and those leaving it. Those of us who have had the privilege of working with our expatriate colleagues are bitterly aware of the true extent of our loss.

For many years doctors who remained here tried hard to overcome the defects of the NHS. They worked far too hard for their own good and the good of their patients. They cut corners with great skill and daring, and improvised with inadequate equipment and facilities. When I left for Canada in 1973 morale in the NHS was good, and there was still a determination to make the NHS work regardless of the difficulties. When I returned in 1977 the situation had deteriorated markedly. Many doctors were counting the days to early retirement, most had given up fighting against the rising tide of indiscipline, erosion of standards, inadequate financing and an over-bearing administration. From the Secretary of State downwards there was an all pervasive air of defeatism.

We are no longer striving to achieve perfection, however slowly and in the face of great difficulties. It has been acknowledged that we cannot look after everybody properly. The retreat has started. The only questions now asked are who will go to the wall, which standards will be sacrificed first and by how much. Discipline, drive and leadership have been eroded and devalued. The workers in the NHS scrabble amongst one another for increased personal reward and status while services to patients suffer.

Although financial reward and status have an enduring importance, the satisfaction of the motivational needs of professional workers is essential for the good of patients and workers. Traditionally the mainspring of medical ethics has been an unqualified requirement that each doctor should do his best for each patient, and that collectively doctors would strive to obtain all that is necessary for the treatment of patients. As public servants doctors have been increasingly frustrated in maintaining adequate standards and are now demoralised.

From idealism to callousness

A young Turk of the Conservative Party recently inveighed against government policy and proclaimed that more money should be spent on health care when the economy picks up and we can afford it. In 1946, in a much harsher economic climate, the founders of the NHS proclaimed that the NHS would provide comprehensive care for everybody who needed it. Although there was an unrealistic view of what could be achieved in practice, that idealism was shared by the providers of health services and the people. That idealism was essential and was responsible for much of the success of the NHS. Its loss has begun to produce a new callousness and selfishness among us that will undermine society.

The victims

The principal victims of a rationing of health services are the old, the chronic sick, the poor and the foolish. We have known of the inadequate services provided for these groups for a long time, particularly for those in institutions. We have been dimly aware of the deprivation of many of these outside institutions. Recently there has been mounting hard evidence of increased illness in these groups. When I visited the Isle of Man, I was shown the fine unit in which people with kidney failure are treated by dialysis. When I asked what percentage of people needing dialysis received it, my question was not understood. When I explained that possibly one third of patients on the mainland were allowed to die, there was horror and incredulity. In that small community the government cannot behave so callously. When a medical member of an English authority resigned in protest against decisions that led to the death of a 54-year-old woman, he was regarded as having over-reacted to an inevitable situation.

Let individuals and communities contribute money and services

From the beginning the NHS has discouraged voluntary effort, public and private philanthropy and self-reliance. In spite of this deadening exclusivity, there is evidence that individuals and communities still want to contribute to their local health services, both in the form of money and services. Failure to encourage this valuable contribution does incalculable harm and creates unnecessary expense. There is also growing evidence of a willingness to pay for services that are rationed by the State. In the short term this may take pressure off the NHS and save public funds in the long run. For many years private practice was a fringe activity for those who wished to spend their money on a luxury service. It is now beginning to assume the characteristics of a black market.

Because most people are not sick at any one time and most people have received adequate care when they needed it, there has been little public awareness of the slow deterioration in the NHS. There has been consistent reluctance to discover the whole costs of the policies adopted and a perfectly natural reluctance on the part of professionals to cause public alarm by drawing attention to inadequacies or poor standards.

Lack of accurate and relevant information accompanied by vigorous propaganda has made it possible for the functioning of health services to be impaired inexorably and slowly over a long period. The longer the delay the bigger will be the difficulty in restoring the morale and efficiency of health service workers.

The time has come when we must count the whole cost of the NHS and then act decisively to cure the ills that afflict services that were once the envy of the world.

XIII
NHS Inflates Social Workers

June Lait

Lecturer in Social Policy at University College, Swansea. Has contributed regularly to the "Daily Telegraph", "World Medicine", and the "Spectator". Author with Colin Brewer of "Can Social Work Survive?" (Maurice Temple Smith, 1980.)

The NHS mis-uses not only doctors but also ancillaries. June Lait maintains that it wastes "social workers" in four activities: in family doctoring, in hospitals, with the disabled and with the mentally ill. And the basic reason is again financial: 'When the taxpayer pays, who cares?' If medical care was paid for by patients themselves, the social workers would probably vanish as medical auxiliaries. The sick would benefit by being treated by qualified nurses and other medical professionals.

Introduction

One of the most daunting aspects of state provision of services we optimistically term "welfare" is the scope afforded for the proliferation of aspiring professions. Buttressed against any market test of effectiveness, they make outrageous claims for status, salary and security of tenure.

There seems to be (or perhaps, post-Thatcher, one should say there *used* to be) a gentlemanly reluctance to question the pretensions of those whose stall is set out under the label "welfare". If one poses the question 'Do social workers do any good?' it is all too easy to be labelled an unsympathetic fascist, grinding the faces of the poor; and most politicians have hitherto been unwilling to incur the risk. This was perhaps a matter of small moment when social service departments had limited functions and relatively small budgets. Now that their annual budgets exceed £800m and they are in the business of enabling 'the greatest possible number of individuals to act reciprocally, giving and receiving service for the well-being of the whole community'. (Seebohm Report, 1968), it matters much more that their pretensions should be examined, their excesses pruned.

State finance and professional pretensions

There is an extensive literature about what constitutes a profession, stressing factors such as a secure knowledge base, a service ethic, extended training, self regulation and licence to practice. It is not the purpose of this essay to assess how far social work can be considered a profession, but to draw attention to ways in which state funding enables social workers to mould their jobs to their own needs, rather than to respond to expressed needs of clients.

It is my contention that the social work functions of social service departments are determined largely by the whims of aspiring professionals, aided and abetted by the reluctance of politicians, and indeed of the general public, to question those who declare their purpose to be the good of mankind, especially when they have managed to acquire a professional training, however bogus. This reluctance would undoubtedly be weakened if the services of social workers were paid for directly, instead of being subsumed in a general levy for "welfare" of one sort or another.

Professions like medicine, which existed before state intervention, and would undoubtedly thrive if state support were withdrawn, are in less danger of providing services satisfying to the providers but useless to the customers than are the artefacts of benevolent bureaucrats. If social work means being kind to the distressed, there have been social workers as long as there has been medicine. By the very nature of their work doctors and nurses involuntarily do "social work" among their patients, but it is only in recent times that the activity has been seen as a basis for a separate profession with a training that excludes medicine but includes all manner of high-sounding activities like fostering: 'the purposeful and ethical application of personal skills in interpersonal relationships directed towards enhancing the personal and social functioning of an individual, family, groups or neighbourhood, which necessarily involves using evidence obtained from practice to help create a social environment conducive to the well-being of all'. This definition of social work was produced by the British Association of Social Workers in furtherance of their view that only "trained" social workers should be allowed to practice. It was laughingly called a "working" definition. Only the taxpayer could be expected to fund such nebulous yet offensively pretentious aspirations.

It seems to me the NHS mis-uses social workers in four activities.

(i) *From Lady Almoners to "interpersonal relationships"*

The association of medicine and social work as a separate activity began with the Lady Almoners, appointed originally to spot fraudulent claims for free treatment in the London teaching hospitals. The first, a Miss Mary Stewart, was appointed to the Royal Free Hospital in 1895. By the inception of the NHS the profession had extended its activities beyond policing, spotting fraud, and assessing charges, and was well and truly launched into the interpersonal relationships business. This was fortunate for medical social workers, as they now called themselves, since a service described as 'free at point of receipt' deprived them at a stroke of their undeniably useful if unprofessionally rewarding financial functions. What it left them with is in some doubt.

Social workers or nurses in hospital?

There is no doubt that illness, and especially admission to hospital can be accompanied by emotional and financial stress. State agencies such as the Supplementary Benefits Commission can relieve some of the financial stress (though whether they are the best agencies to do so is quite another matter), and medical social workers can refer patients to these agencies. To do this effectively requires a telephone principally; it is doubtful in the extreme whether it requires a degree followed by a postgraduate training in social work, the present preferred qualification for medical social workers.

Emotional stress is something else, and I doubt whether anyone without medical knowledge (or possibly *anyone at all*) is well placed to understand the conditions giving rise to it. This knowledge social workers do *not* have. Yet in our odd state-funded scheme of things they are paid substantially more than the nurses on the wards for an exceedingly dubious expertise. Nurses, in regular and intimate contact with their patients, can be the best of counsellors if they have time to spare.

(ii) *Why do GPs use social workers?*

Social workers are sometimes attracted to general practices, where their function is to deal with the social and emotional problems that fall outside the remit of the GP. GPs who have social workers are usually enthusiastic about them. This is hardly surprising, as they cost the practice nothing directly: their substantial salaries are paid by the local authority who seconds them to the GP. Another and cheaper variant is for GPs to employ volunteer counsellors, and a report of the Royal College of GPs finds them acceptable.

An interesting research project is at present under way at the Institute of Psychiatry, seeking to assess the special nature of the contribution social workers make. It would be a betrayal of confidence to pre-empt the findings, which are not yet complete, but it would not be an exaggeration to say that the researchers are doubtful whether the popularity of social workers with GPs depends on particular skills, or whether they just value another pair of hands provided at the public expense. If, as I suspect, it is the latter, a graduate with a postgraduate training makes an expensive auxiliary. But then, when the taxpayer pays, who cares?

And when an expert in 'interpersonal relationships, creating environments conducive to the wellbeing of all', is in question, who dares? (As a matter of fact Dr Colin Brewer and I do in a new book, *Can Social Work Survive?* (Maurice Temple Smith, 1980) and we hope you'll read it).

(iii) *Can social workers judge disablement?*

The Chronically Sick and Disabled Persons Act of 1970 recommends to local authority social service departments many benevolent activities they could undertake on behalf of the handicapped, such as the provision of free telephones, meals on wheels, and issuing stickers for cars that advertise the driver's incapacity. It is well known that the variations between local authorities in such provisions are very wide. Provoked by a recent personal experience, I wonder whether the cost of administering these benefits may not outweigh any possible benefit to the recipients, or at least those few recipients who get them. I also find a matter of great concern the assumption underlying the Chronically Sick and Disabled Person's Act that *anyone* unlucky enough to be ill may also be unlucky enough to require the ministrations of a social worker.

Unlike the doctor, the social worker comes uninvited to assess eligibility for various benefits, though how she can do this without medical knowledge is a puzzle. In practice, she can't. A close relation of mine receives mobility allowance from the Department of Health and Social Security, a cash sum and exemption from car tax awarded after a rigorous medical examination by a specially appointed doctor (not the patient's own). Only people unable to walk qualify for mobility allowance. The "disabled" label, seemingly far more common, allows parking on yellow lines, and is issued not by the DHSS but by the Social Services Department. To obtain it one must fill in a form, obtain a certificate from one's doctor, and unless one is very determined, submit to a visit from a social worker. The form we completed had space for signature by social worker, senior social worker, and area social services officer.

What possible grounds are there for giving discretion to such people in medical matters, apart from proliferating administration to find work for people unqualified for anything better? It is no surprise to me to hear that "Disabled" labels are for sale in many parts of the country, and that police view the whole affair with cynicism.

(iv) *Are social workers competent in mental illness?*

In mental illness social workers have an ill-defined role and, in my opinion, a lack of competence. The assessment of mental illness is a skilled matter, its treatment difficult and of doubtful outcome. There is at present a vogue for care of the mentally ill "in the community", a phrase used hopefully rather than accurately by many social workers. Much social work training stresses the disadvantages of institutional care, no doubt with good reason, but the distaste for it amounts quite frequently to a foolish, sometimes dangerous, and frequently callous determination to subject people whose mental health is frail to the rigours of living in a community which frequently rejects them.

Few doctors of my acquaintance wish to institutionalise their patients without good cause, or incarcerate them longer than necessary. And how long "necessary" is only doctors (if anyone) are qualified to judge. Many report exasperation and alarm at the activities of social workers, indoctrinated in enthusiasm for "the community". Having arranged the transfer from an institution they get bored with the wearisome details of coping with the patient afterwards. Many patients land back in institutions damaged by their experience of a rejecting community.

Conclusion

In summary, the four areas of social work interaction with medicine are in hospital, in general practice, in work with the disabled, and the mentally ill. In none of these fields have social workers a special competence which justifies their high salaries *vis-a-vis* nurses or typists. In all of them they are at best regarded as medical auxiliaries, or minor bureaucrats. Only the elastic purse of the compulsorily benevolent taxpayer permits them to posture as anything else. In a free market society they would probably vanish without trace, and the sick be none the worse. Since responsibility would then be firmly with the competent, I expect the sick would do better.

XIV
Blind Alleys in "Health Education"

Digby C. Anderson

Researched into the practicalities of health education at the
University of Nottingham. Tutored the Health Education Certificate course and researched into the justifications and arguments
of sociologists and social interventionalists for his doctorate in
sociology. Has edited a book on Health Education and written
numerous articles. Editor of a series on Strategies of Professional
Development and "The Ignorance of Social Intervention" (Croom
Helm, 1980). Author of "Evaluating Curricular Proposals"
(Croom Helm), a criticism of Schools Council curricular projects.

As "free" medicine and its chronic financial anaemia crowds out
the really sick by the not-really-sick, raises costs, reduces quality,
cuts out services, provokes the reluctant taxpayer, subjects medicine
to predatory strikes and party politics, there is hopeful attention to
"health education" as a way to reduce the demands on overworked
doctors and nurses. If the British will not pay more in taxes for a
better NHS perhaps they can be persuaded to look after their health
themselves. Is this a way out for the NHS? Digby Anderson says
the health educators themselves must be educated out of unprofessional attitudes, inefficient methods and hopeless dreams.
And they should accept that the public may want health care and
education to pass from the State to private organisation.

Introduction

Some people visit schools and inform 14-year-old girls of the awful consequences of wearing high-heeled shoes. That, say the health educationists, is *not* what health education is about. Other people design colourful posters and inventive television commercials about flies and running. That, say health educationists, is only a small part of what health education is about.

Who are the "health educators"?

Health educationists currently define their work both differently and more generously than these activities. Health education for them is a range of aims, agents, problems and techniques. It may include:

1) The *dietician* informing and motivating the obese patient to help him to understand and organise his diet more successfully.
2) The *health visitor* educating expectant mothers for parenthood.
3) The *youth worker* counselling adolescents about difficulties in personal relationships.
4) The *health education officer* running a stop-smoking clinic or a local campaign.
5) The *teacher* using "role-play" to help her pupils make more mature and responsible decisions about themselves and others.
6) A *group* pressuring for change in pollution or occupational legislation.

Health educationists represent their work as a concern for health, not merely for disease-avoidance; as influencing attitudes, "climates of opinion" and behaviour, not "just" giving information; as communication through text, television and telephone as well as through talk in clinics; as using instructional, pedagogic, advertising, group work, behaviour modification and counselling techniques more than medical accounts; as concerned with education for the "better" use of NHS services, with personal relationships, community development, ethnic minorities, with mental and social well being, with "lifestyle", and with patient education rather than with warnings. (A fuller description is in D. C. Anderson, *Health Education in Practice*, Croom Helm, 1979.)

Although health educators are keen to involve everyone in this work, it remains true that the staff involved consists largely of NHS or LEA workers such as doctors, nurses, teachers, health visitors, social workers and environmental health officers.

What are they all doing?

The health educator is then increasingly defining his role as persuading certain of these workers to increase and improve the educational aspects of their work and as providing resources to assist this increase and improvement. He sees his job with such staff as persuasion, support and co-ordination. These supporting, persuading, co-ordinating bodies are, centrally, the Health Education Council (created in 1968 and funded almost entirely by central government at around £4,000,000) and, at AHA level, 342 Health Education Officers (1978). Supplementing their efforts are two Schools' Council projects, masters' (Chelsea College) diploma, certificate and in-service courses; three professional organisations; half a dozen English research projects; the Scottish Health Education Unit; many more individual researches and several journals. From the point of view of the NHS, health education can be conceived of as a pressure group which wants to change workers' training and practices and to increase the resources allocated to "educational" tasks rather than others.

All this suggests a picture of health education as a busy and varied activity. To this it should be added that both the business and the variety have grown enormously in the last ten years. the budget of the organisation which the Health Education Council replaced, the Central Council for Health Education, was under £60,000 in its last year (1967/68). And with more money has come the interest in different techniques, agents and settings for health education. Certainly it must be stressed that the Health Education Council has taken a sensible and successful path in the last decade, in spending its money on a variety of matters, methods and men. Since little was known about explicit health education, such an open and experimental policy made good sense. But there comes a time for experiments to be "written up" and for results to be inspected to see not whether health education should continue but which aspects of it should continue and which should not. I suggest the time is now for health educators to step back and assess the state of their work. Having done this they could take two positive steps forward.

High time to ask what good they are doing

The time is now for assessment largely because of financial considerations . . . Health educators may be faced not only with cuts in their own budgets but also with cuts in the budgets of the NHS and LEA staff who do the health education fieldwork. There are at least four ways in which health educators could respond to the event (rather than the promise) of contracting state support.

(i) *"Fighting the cuts": unprofessional and inefficient*

First, they could adopt a trade union attitude and "look after the membership". This might involve "fighting the cuts" to the last minute, then doing a hasty, unmethodic and inelegant retreat in which all sorts of services were trimmed but the personnel left intact.

This seems to be the current attitude of the teachers' union. It is essentially cutting for the professionals' rather than for the clients' benefit, though it is usually wrapped up in formulae which *totally* and thus implausibly equate the two. 'We are not trying to keep our jobs for our own sakes but for the sakes of our clients'. Such an attitude is thoroughly unprofessional. And it is inefficient because it ignores the logical and practical interrelationships between staff and non-staff "assets".

(ii) *Deciding "need": not for health educators to judge*

Secondly, services could be cut on the basis of "need". The work which caters for the biggest or most urgent "need" is the work retained. There are a number of objections to this approach. Most obviously the health and personal services have never been very good at explaining or justifying priorities in times of expansion let alone contraction. "Need" has typically been decided by the professional rather than the client, and in health education there has been a mania for collecting as many as possible causes to follow, clients to "compassionate" and techniques to adopt.

That mania is plausible in times of experiment, but not very useful now. To it has been added an argument, borrowed, I suspect, from sociology, which inter-relates all these needs, causes, problems and clients. It suggests that in social life all problems occur within familial biographical, community, attitudinal, ethnic and overall socio-political contexts. The object of those who follow such ideas is to widen rather than contain the problems they address. But they are not well equipped for finding economic solutions to discrete needs. An enterprise which has been trying to explore as many aspects of problems as possible and is showing increasing signs of succumbing to the notion that everything is related to everything else is not in a good position to be precise and modest. For the practical issue in a world of scarce resources is not whether one *can* see many aspects of a problem but whether one *must* see them in order to solve it. (Further discussed in *Irony*, Harvester Press, 1980.)

(iii) *An incentive to realism*

This reasoning suggests a third heretical reaction to unavoidable contraction in resources. Economies could be welcomed as an incentive to practical self-assessment and realism. Health educators could turn contraction into a step forward by looking back over the last decade, over the many causes, campaigns, techniques, aims and agents, and taking a delight in separating the ideal from the possible, the illusory from the practical.

They could at last rid themselves of definitions of "health" which include all aspects of well-being, and definitions of "education" which include all forms of communication. They could abandon working with professionals whose involvement has not proved useful. They could abandon clients who do not seem to profit from their intervention. They could abandon working in unproductive settings. They could fasten on the tasks which can be done, and which have been done successfully, and cease to gaze wistfully at those, so much more alluring, which are interesting but impractical. They could use methods suited to handle the target, but no bigger.

Not least, they could accept that health education is about changing people. Those who find this distasteful and would rather 'facilitate environments wherein people can make their own health decisions' could realise that their techniques do not become any more practical by being nicer. Changing people is difficult whether it is done directly or indirectly, in a democratic or in a manipulative way. Since the work is difficult, the objective should be not to try and find as *many* people to change as possible, not to worry because one cannot get at everyone, but to find a few changes which really are necessary, technically possible within existing resources and settings and, not least, appreciated by the client, patient or audience.

(iv) *The state is not the only source of funds*

The fourth, tentative and totally heretical reaction to the contraction of state support, both for health education and the NHS in general, would be for health educationists to re-appraise their attitude to the state and private enterprise.

While is would be unrealistic to talk of anything so coherent as a "position" of health educators towards the state, it is clear that health education is permeated with statist assumptions based on the notion that only the state can provide or finance it. First, there is often an antagonistic attitude to private enterprise as such in any form. Many health educators would wish in particular to "control" the marketing and advertising of such industries as supply alcoholic drinks and tobacco. Secondly, most health educators act as if the NHS is a permanent fixture. They have not even started

86

to think about how they might adapt themselves to an expanded private sector. This failure is bizarre not only because an expanded private sector is a real possibility, but because some forms of private medical care have health education potential.

It is odd that health educators, with their emphasis on people making their own health decisions and taking responsibility for their own health, should wish to shield people from the financial consequences of their decisions about health-related behaviour. It is odd that when they talk so much of 'need' they should not use, or even think of using, demand as an indication of it. It is odd that some health educators should encourage the state to link benefits to behaviour (e.g. maternity benefits to attendance at ante-natal classes) but no health educator is currently urging the benefits of market incentives.

Consider for instance one of the problems health educators find both in transmitting information and in modifying behaviour. They are aware that the rewards and penalties of decisions related to health often follow some years after. They know that alcoholism, cancer, dental caries and many others take time to develop from drinking, smoking and eating sugar. They know that distant consequences are not perceived as real. And so they try to find short-term disincentives, such as in posters which show the girl friend refusing to kiss the tobacco-smelling boy. What better regular short-term disincentive could there be than a medical insurance premium as a financial inducement to avoid harmful habits related to behaviour; smoking, drinking, over-eating . . .?

Private health education growing

Health educators could also note that there is already not only a private health sector but a private health education sector. It is an ideologically mixed bag of private enterprise, voluntary groups, radical medico-political groups, and trusts. It includes Weight Watchers, the National Childbirth Trust (for ante-natal help), the Keep-Fit industry, Women's "consciousness raising" groups, alternative medicine organisations, voluntary groups for sufferers from many illnesses, mental health organisations, books sold for profit and profitable to the reader, and so on. Clearly some people *can* take care of their health without having to be told, advised, warned or "facilitated" by tax-paid officials. Clearly some people *can* organise effective health education programmes and appreciated health education programmes without state assistance. Indeed it is arguable that in technical innovations these non-state bodies have been ahead of the full-time "official" government-employed health educators.

Some health education is of course based on epidemiological data about national or regional patterns of "need", and the programmes which issue from it may have no easily identifiable individual beneficiary. Some health education is very much a long-term business and is for people not yet able to "demand" it for themselves. But even if these are set aside, there is still a large amount of health education which is aimed at fairly short-term help for individual and discrete identifiable groups and persons. Given the obvious practicality of some private health education, the emphasis on personal responsibility, the desirability of short-term reinforcements, and the practical exigencies of contraction in state finance health, educators face a challenge to justify their nearly exclusive reliance on state assistance.

Initiating tax-funded "causes" of serving the public prepared to pay

Many would be reluctant to do so. For some, perhaps, a life initiating interesting "causes" is more congenial than one responding to demand in a competitive market. For others the moral stance of much health education has to be protected from the contamination of the market. For yet others health education is a front for compensatory intervention, yet one more way of championing the reluctant urban poor. But for most an unquestioning trust in statism is, I suspect, an occupational hazard – something that comes with the job. They were never taught to think it could be otherwise. They should think of that possibility now.

For if health educators claim to offer so many benefits to the public, to organisations and to their fellow health professionals; if they really have the key to better public and personal health, more effective communication for health workers, a healthier, more productive industry: why are they not prepared to see if people will *pay* for these benefits.

XV
The NHS is Inadequate for Industry and Trade Unions

Arthur Seldon

Will the NHS suit British industry and its employees for all time? Will they be content to accept its deteriorating services no matter the delays, inconveniences, disruptions to the working life? Loyalty to a long-cherished hope that the NHS would be able to provide rising standards and quality of service explain why the first radical breach was delayed until 1980. Since 1 January a collective agreement between employers and a trade union has taken 40,000 wage-earners (and, if they wish, for a small cost, their families) out of the NHS into private medicine. This essay crystallises the acerbic doctrinal dispute that has broken out between trade union leaders, and emphasises its significance for the future of the NHS, since there is no reason to suppose the agreement will be the last in British industry.

Introduction

A severe charge against the state control of medicine is that its employees will form an organised bloc united to defend their jobs in the *status quo* whatever its service to the public, and to resist reform whatever the preference of the public.

This apotheosis of reaction has predictably come to pass. The unions want more tax money for higher pay for more jobs. Everything else is secondary. And they hope to get their way with government because they can strike or otherwise damage the nation's health services. But before long technical change and innovation make possible new or improved services that government cannot suppress, even to avoid confrontation with the unions.

Screening for electricians

Such an innovation is screening. It enables employers of expensive labour to detect early symptoms of incapacity. They can then take action by prompt treatment without the costly delays of the NHS.

The electrical contractors place large numbers of their skilled craftsmen on building sites where accidents and fatalities are second only to mining. The absence of one or two trained staff can disrupt a working team or a whole contract. So the employers discussed an "early warning" system with the trade union representatives on the Joint Industry Board. The employers spoke through the Electrical Contractors Association (ECA), led by the Chairman of its Industrial Relations Department, Michael Stothers. The union is the Electrical, Electronic, Telecommunications and Plumbing Union (EEPTU), led by its General Secretary, Frank Chapple.

The ECA was concerned about the health of its workforce and the prevention of accidents. The EETPU was concerned about improving the working conditions of its members. The two agreed on a scheme for three-yearly screening of 40,000 electricians. If indicated, early or immediate treatment would follow. Both services had to be arranged outside the NHS because the NHS does not supply "free" regular screening and it does not supply immediate or early treatment. So both services were arranged by private insurance through the British United Provident Association (BUPA). The scheme began in January 1980.

Trade union leaders defend NHS, attack competition

Uproar! The arrangement was announced in August 1979. By the time of the TUC Conference in September the familiar and predictable accusations had been well-honed. Mr Bernard Dix of the National Union of Public Employees attacked the principle. 'We don't care how you buy privilege, whether you are an oil sheik or a trade unionist, we want it out.' 'We' are presumably his union. 'Out' means they want the law to prevent *anyone* from spending more on his health than the state can persuade *everyone* to pay in taxes. Mr Albert Spanswick of the Confederation of Health Service Employees said: 'If we put a stop to . . . . these insurance deals . . . . among ourselves now in a friendly way, the private sector will wither away.' Again the 'we' who shall lay down where the sick shall be treated is the union – or its officials. So the NHS is a very *syndicalist* rather than a *public* service. And there was the echo of Marx in the notion of the private sector 'withering away' (except that Marx said the state would wither away under socialism, perhaps his most damaging bad judgement).

90

Perhaps unexpectedly the EETPU's spokesman at the TUC Conference (and at the October 1979 Labour Party Conference), Eric Hammond, was not intimidated. He not only defended the arrangement as part of the time-honoured function of a union, classically defined by the Webbs, to improve the working conditions of its members. He counter-attacked the critics: some trade union leaders, he asserted, took their medical problems 'behind the Iron Curtain' (*The Sun*, 5 September 1979). 'The English had a world wide fame for hypocrisy, but our critics' attitude must take all the prizes' (*Daily Express,* 5 September). 'Many other groups are seeking similar deals' (*Daily Telegraph,* 5 September).

Another trade union leader was caught in the cross-fire when he tried to combine loyalty to the NHS with the health of trade unionist. Mr Sidney Weighall of the National Union of Railwaymen explained: 'This [Manor House Hospital] is a very different case from the organisations which enable the wealthy to jump queues. The NUR and other unions have deeds of covenant which provide the hospital with much of its funds . . .' (*Daily Telegraph*, 5 September). And Mr Moss Evans of the Transport and General Workers Union weighed in with his support.

But if it is proper for some trade unions to contribute outside the NHS to the upkeep of a hospital for their private treatment, why not all eleven million trade unionists – and their wives and children?

Trade union leader attacks NHS, defends private medicine

A few days after the TUC Conference the EETPU General Secretary reinforced his spokesman by what must be described as an historic article in a mass newspaper read by manual workers and their wives (*News of the World,* 9 September). Perhaps because he is of outstanding intelligence and stands by his principles, or because he is a former Communist who knows all the arguments (and the false claims) in the century-old case for state control of everything, or because he dislikes humbug, his unexpected counter-attack on an ark of the collectivist/Labour covenant will rank in the annals of trade union history. It was an uncompromising defence of his union's agreement with the employers, a withering assault on other trade union leaders, and a root and branch questioning and rejection of the claim for the NHS as an exclusive state monopoly. (Editor's italics in following extracts.)

He spoke of 'hypocrisy' in the trade union movement. He denounced 'holier-than thou' union leaders who had attacked his 'private health treatment deal'. Whatever the criticisms it would stand because it 'made good sense'.

His union supported the NHS (a logical error in view of his later criticism) but 'as inefficiency grows, along with the waiting-list for treatment, *so will grow private health care*'. But if private medicine spreads, I must interpose, what becomes of the comprehensive NHS?

Moreover, it could 'justifiably' be argued that private care 'could ease the strain' on the NHS. So the NHS is *not* comprehensive.

He accused his critics of failing to show how his scheme could 'weaken' the NHS, which was already 'under considerable strain' financially and physically in its huge waiting lists.

He then listed five cases of 'hypocrisy':

1. There was no condemnation of Liverpool women who accepted open heart surgery in a private hospital because it was not available in the NHS.

2. There was no condemnation of industrial disputes that delayed the building of new NHS hospitals and so deprived the public of medical services.
3. The building unions have never considered preferential treatment for NHS hospitals or other state projects.
4. Many politicians and trade union *leaders* have long had private treatment. The row had broken out only when *rank and file* union members were offered the same services.
5. There was no condemnation of the preferential treatment for NHS member unions and their relatives. The row had broken out only when non-NHS EETPU members had been offered the same 'preferential treatment'.

Doctors and nurses would want preferential treatment for their families in queues or waiting lists. The row had broken out because 'blue-collar workers' were to receive the same treatment as 'white-collar and managerial working groups". The same accusing note – that it was the NHS unions (or rather their officials) that were defending privilege – continued remorsely throughout the whole article.

Mr Chapple repudiated the charge that the EETPU had ensured the downfall of members of the NHS unions. 'The death knell sounded for them' in the 1974 reorganisation. The four-tier administration, 'overseen by an overstaffed DHSS administration', was a handicap under which no public institution would prosper. Yet, he added, every union except the EETPU had advocated no redundancy, thus *'ensuring the retention of this inefficient system'*. The major NHS unions had a vested interest in this policy: 'their growth in membership (since 1974) had not been inconsiderable'.

"Patient" – electricians' union leader condemns NHS union leader

And then this damaging attack on COHSE and NUPE:
1. They would be unlikely to support measures to help 'the tottering NHS' because 'their strength comes from its inadequacies'.
2. 'They have added to the NHS problems through their industrial disputes for higher wages.'

And the final rejection: 'Now they have the cheek to assert it is my agreement which will undermine the [NHS] service'.

If the NHS deterioration continues, 'people, trade unionists or not, will be forced to obtain outside treatment, *irrespective of principles or costs'*. So much for the vain wishful thinking that the sanctity of the "free" NHS would be put before individual health.

Humbug on private beds: if you can't join 'em, beat 'em

Mr Chapple had views on revising the sacred NHS "free" principle: people who made no contributions to its running costs should be restricted. (Presumably this meant tourists or other overseas visitors.) Then the opposite is also true. It is only a short step to argue that the more the contribution, the better the service should be, as a Labour leader (now a peer) argued some years ago as the way to raise more funds for the NHS.

And then an attack on another form of humbug. NHS workers have long complained against doctors with patients in private beds. Mr Chapple's reply: '. . . . the biggest complaint of NHS workers . . . . was that they were not sharing in the payments . . . . If there had been some form of bonus arrangement . . . . there would probably have been fewer complaints and possibly no campaign for the removal of private beds'.

Finally, the challenge to the practicability of a universal 'free' NHS. The critics' views were 'illusory': 'They came largely from those with soft jobs in the system or from demagogues who wish to limit choice, [who] want to dictate who will have treatment, where and when – and with themselves usually first.'

Moreover, they were fooling their followers: 'These demagogues will never stop trying to delude the labour movement and the British people into a non-competitive society where no-one seeks to beat the other man.'

Could such a society exist?

'Experience shows it is very unlikely. Certainly it does not exist anywhere else in the world . . . .'

Why is this inter-union quarrel important?

This is the judgment not of a proselyte blinded by dogma, but of a trade union leader convinced by experience. Logic led him from a defence of his union in improving the position of his members to a radical questioning of the very foundations of the NHS itself: the great achievement of the "labour movement" and the "envy of the world".

Other British industries have occupations in which work is liable to accident, in which screening can detect, and early treatment remove, conditions that cause accident-proneness.

Frank Chapple was the first leader of a union to put his members before the dogma of a dying experiment in state medicine. There is no reason to suppose he will be the last.

XVI
NHS Medicine is Infected by Egalitarian politics

Ivor Jones

Born 1919 on Tyneside. Educated Grammar School, University College, Nottingham and Newcastle-upon-Tyne Medical School. House surgeon to Professor of Surgery. General practice near Sunderland. Became involved in medical politics in 1952 when elected to Representative Body of BMA; 1954, elected to BMA council; Chairman, Private Practice Committee 1958–1970; Member of BMA negotiating team 1964 to 1970; Member Royal Commission Evidence Committee (1957-60); Chairman, BMA Medical Services Review Committee, 1958-61; Member of Council 1954-70; Chairman, Committee on Health Services Financing, 1968-70; County practice in Wiltshire from 1971 until retirement in 1979.

A "hidden cost" of the NHS that its supporters keep well out of sight is the subjection of medicine to party politics. In this essay Ivor Jones, for some years a BMA negotiator with government on the pay and other conditions of family doctors, reveals the political factors in medical policy since 1948. He talks of the broken promises, the resistence to change, the consolidation of power by politicians and bureaucrats, the cynical subordination of the health of the people to political dogma. He also strongly condemns the BMA for flinching at the truth and pigeon-holing a report in 1970 that pointed to reforms now seen as dangerously neglected.

Introduction

Few people now question that the NHS is desperately short of money. The recent tightening of cash limits by the Minister of Health has emphasised a trend extending over thirty years and has brought protests from health authorities unable to fulfil objectives imposed by the NHS Acts in prevention, diagnosis and treatment of disease. There will be many more protests. The solution requires consideration of the attitude taken by Government and by doctors in similar crises of financial stringency since the NHS was created.

The initial mistake

The final impetus to the creation of the NHS was provided by the Medical Planning Commission of the BMA in 1940 and the Beveridge Report of 1942, which postulated the necessity for:

> a health service providing full preventive and curative treatment of every kind to every citizen, without exceptions, without remuneration limit and without an economic barrier at any point to delay recourse to it.

The NHS Act of 1946 established it as a duty of the Minister of Health:

> to promote the establishment of a comprehensive health service designed to secure improvement in the physical and mental health of the people and the prevention, diagnosis and treatment of illness, and for that purpose to provide or secure the effective provision of services.

In fulfilling the duty imposed by Parliament, successive Conservative and Labour governments have chosen to *provide* rather than to *secure the effective provision* of health services. They have created the three causes of recurring and mounting trouble: they

1. provided through a very centralised machinery under the control of a Minister;
2. financed the services almost exclusively by *taxation;* and
3. made the services almost entirely *free at the point of use.*

Within months it became clear to the Treasury that an initial estimate of £265m for the annual cost of the NHS would be exceeded by at least half. The embarrassment caused panic in the Government, and led to the 1949 Cripps budget erosion of the original concept of providing optimal care for all, by specifying a ceiling of £400m per year and provision of as much free care as was possible within it. There is no evidence that the Government gave any serious consideration to change in the financial structure of the NHS. Ministers retained faith in the mistaken forecast of Beveridge that the size of the bill would fall as the nation became healthier.

Although the sum allocated has risen over the years with changes in costs and in the value of money, and we are devoting a higher percentage of GNP to the NHS than in 1949, the principle of the Cripps decree has been perpetuated by successive governments. Real growth in health services has been of minor order; it is attributable to scientific advances as distinct from improvements in organisation or finance.

Another mistake: doctors' pay

Government made another miscalculation. Before inauguration of the NHS two committees chaired by Sir Will Spens had been established to advise on the incomes to be paid to family doctors and hospital consultants. Their recommendations had been accepted by the government and the BMA but were expressed in 1939 values of money. Spens did not know precisely when the NHS would be launched and 'left it to others' to adjust his figures in the light of changes in the value of money and in other comparable incomes. Government initially applied a betterment factor of 20 per cent to Spens' figures, thus ignoring his criteria. Discussions between the Government and the BMA soon reached *impasse*. The issue, for family doctors, was referred to Mr Justice Danckwerts as arbitrator. He found for the doctors, criticised the Government, and awarded a betterment factor of 100 per cent. Corresponding changes had to be made in the pay of hospital staff. The cost of the NHS was raised substantially.

Successive Governments have been acutely embarrassed by the cost of the NHS ever since. In 1952, after the Danckwerts adjudication, the Prime Minister, Winston Churchill, informed Parliament that the Government would never submit to independent arbitration again. In the event, the new Prime Minister, Harold Macmillion, was compelled in 1957 to submit the issue of doctors' pay to a Royal Commission, having first refused to discuss or consider a claim for an increase of at least 24 per cent on pay, unchanged since 1952. It was made clear to the BMA by Mr Macmillan that the Government, despite earlier acceptance of the Spens reports and the Danckwerts award, did not accept any obligation as employer to take into account changes in the value of money or in comparable incomes. Later he claimed that no opinion on the merits of the claim had been implied, and that economic circumstances made it impossible to consider the matter. (What an example to set for other employers!)

The 1957-1960 Royal Commission, chaired by Sir Harry Pilkington, found no difficulty in establishing the change in the value of money, but was handicapped by the absence of reliable information on the changes in comparable incomes. Within months of appointment the Commission instigated modest increases in pay to be made immediately on account. In the final Pilkington report of February 1960, the Government was censured for failing to carry out the recommendations of Spens and reminded that:

> if the nation wants the benefits [of an NHS] it must accept the cost, provide the means to ascertain the facts and to do financial justice, neither less nor more, to those who work in that service.

In raising doctors' remuneration by approximately 23 per cent the Commission advised that an independent Review Body be created to determine doctors' pay and that its recommendations 'must only very rarely and for most obviously compelling reasons be rejected'.

Prime Minister, Royal Commission and Review Bodies

Government implemented the Royal Commission's recommendations in 1960, but by 1966 under Harold Wilson was back to the old tricks with a new one called 'phasing', under which it accepted the findings of the Review Body 'in principle' but delayed full implementation. This new style obviously appealed to Edward Heath, who perpetuated the habit, bolstered it wih an "incomes policy" for Harold Wilson to continue when returned to power in 1974. Injustice to doctors continued until Margaret Thatcher implemented the most recent Review Body recommendations in June 1980. No sooner was this done than doubts began to be raised in official quarters in regard to the position for the future.

Long ago the NHS, despite many obvious defects, had become a sacred cow to the Labour Party and a political requirement in the minds of Conservatives. Perhaps because of this philosophic dogma and electoral tactics no thought was given by either Party to the desirability of reconsidering the 1948 decision to finance medical care by taxation and to exclude a pricing mechanism.

Relations between Government and the BMA were soured by the humiliation of ministers and civil servants first by Danckwerts, then by Pilkington. Though discussions continued between representatives of doctors and the Ministry of Health, the stock reply to any suggestions by the BMA for improvement in the NHS was that no money could be made available. Nor would Ministers contemplate any modification in financing "the Service" to raise more money than could be raised by taxation.

Political resistance to change

No one who has taken part in discussions with the Ministry of Health, as I have done, could be under any illusion about the vehemence of resistance to change. The financial structure of the NHS, though presented as a sound economic investment, was not primarily designed to that end. It derived from a different and in some ways conflicting doctrine of *equality* – and the purpose was to ensure that, regardless of the quality of the service, all men and women should have a free and equal access to all types of medical care. The structure has been perpetuated by the political desire to control through a virtual monopoly at the lowest cost to the Treasury. This obsession of the civil servant mind is revealed throughout the last thirty years in numerous ways. Three examples are:

1. Despite Aneurin Bevan's promise in launching the NHS that citizens would be able to use the services for which they were to pay in taxes and national insurance contributions 'in whole or in part' people who choose – and make sacrifices – to obtain family doctor advice privately are denied the drugs necessary in treatment on the same terms as NHS patients.
2. Governments have, despite requests to do otherwise, insisted on remunerating doctors either by salary or by capitation fees – the two most undesirable methods conceivable. But they carry the advantage *to government* of facilitating very accurate budgeting of the cost of an open-ended commitment to the community; and they limit the clerical work load of the doctors. But, at a high cost, they impair the doctor-patient relationship by providing no incentive to effort. And they fail to reflect the differences in either quantity or quality of work performed. The only system which makes for the best service by the doctor to the patient is payment by unit of service – the system which has always been refused.
3. The Ministry of Health has always resented that it had to concede the continuation of a limited number of pay-beds in many of the hospitals taken over in 1948. During the recent years it has succeeded in considerably reducing their number, so that it is now often impossible for people willing to pay twice (in effect) for their hospital care to find the means of doing so. I remember Richard Crossman, then Secretary of State, admitting to me in 1966 that this attitude was quite illogical because it deprived the NHS of a source of income, but that to do otherwise would negate socialist principles.

Government prevents people paying more for medical care

Today most of our hospitals are around 75 years old and many have become quite unsuitable for the practice of modern medicine. They are inadequately staffed at all medical levels and are inadequately equipped. Why? – because they cannot afford to be otherwise: because they are limited to the finance which government is capable of raising through taxation.

New hospital building throughout Europe has been on a vastly larger scale than in Britain, where professional advice is ignored because government lacks the money it will not allow people to pay in ways they prefer. The situation is deteriorating to the point that hospital authorities are openly protesting that they are unable to maintain *essential* services, let alone contemplate *optimal* standards. To the community it presents long and lengthening waiting lists for both consultation and treatment in face of the scientific desirability of increasing specialist advice in the practice of modern medicine.

Most people are aware of deficiences in the NHS. These deficiences all require money to correct them. The money is denied not because people do not wish to provide it, or because they cannot afford to supply it, but because of *government insistence on finance by taxation* and rigid control. We are spending a smaller proportion of national income on health care than before World War II (then about 6 per cent). Nothing has advanced since Douglas Jay announced that the man in Whitehall knows best.

NHS behind medical care in other countries

Ten years ago, in compiling an international league table of health statistics Sir George Godber, a vociferous defender of 'the achievements of the NHS', could place Britain only eighth among developed nations of the world. In 1948, we were probably second. Using the same criteria today, we would vie with Italy for bottom place. *(Italy is discussed in Essay XXIII. – Ed.)*

Yet the community as a whole remains complacent, continues to rejoice in the delusion that "free medical services" are not exposed to a pricing mechanism of any kind, and fails to relate these features to the deficiences about which it grumbles with an ever-louder voice.

One has only to observe, as the World Health Organisation has done, the other countries which are achieving better results. All are devoting a considerably higher proportion of their national income to health services. But they are relying much more on direct charges and voluntary and compulsory systems of health insurance rather than taxation as their principal source of finance.

As Professor J. M. Buchanan of the USA noted when he was here some years ago, 'citizens as taxpayers are not prepared to provide collectively as much free care as they demand individually'. Socialists (in all political parties) may regret this truth, but cannot change it. People are willing and eager to expend more of their money on the health of themselves and their families than they are willing to contribute to the care of others.

Government and BMA flinched from truth

Forget the old lie that our NHS is the envy of the world. It is not. All have been to look and none have copied *(except Italy – on paper. Essay XXI – Ed.)*. The gap between our performance and that of comparable nations is widening every year. On the present basis it would cost the equivalent of an additional 25p in the pound on the standard rate of income tax to bridge it. Enough said.

The BMA, under presure from doctors all over the country, set up a committe of inquiry into the NHS, under my chairmanship, in 1967. Their report, published in 1970, demonstrated beyond any possible doubt that there is little prospect of tax revenue matching the increasing cost of providing health services at even the *current* inadequate quality. And there is no prospect that tax revenue can ever provide the *rising* standards which science makes possible and which should be the aspiration of us all.

The validity of these conclusions has never been seriously challenged. But they were unwelcome to government and, for this reason, unwelcome to some of the BMA hierarchy who were more concerned with their own personal ambitions than with the exposition of truth or the welfare of the British people. Despite a notable lack of BMA effort to promote sale, this report was soon sold out, though it has never been reprinted.

The report proposed that the role of taxation should be limited to public health services and preventative medicine, capital expenditure on hospitals and general practice buildings, medico-welfare services including subsidy of the chronic sick and the indigent, and research and education. But medical care by personal physician, District General Hospital and Accident Hospital care and the treatment of acute mental illness should be financed by direct charges buttressed by flexible health insurance schemes. For these services there is no reason to preclude competition between the State and private agencies, which could stimulate each other.

The only way out

Such arrangements would not only encourage people to make better provision for themselves than government is ever likely to make for them. They would also foster higher standards of service by doctors and hospitals that would find it impossible to reduce either quality or availability of service without reducing their own incomes – a powerful deterrent to bad behaviour. And I think that waiting lists of all kinds would be sharply reduced in a very short time.

The practice of medicine in Britain was politicised in 1948 and has been imprisoned be egalitarian jailers ever since. Margaret Thatcher's government gives some hope of relief, but the way ahead will be a rough road leading to a goal which cannot be reached without stimulus and support from British doctors and the British people, who have no desire to perpetuate a future as the Cinderellas of Europe and the western world.

So long as the present financial structure of the NHS is maintained, the government must either impose considerable increase in taxation, which would be disastrous, or face a deterioration in the quality of medical care, which would be unacceptable to the British people. There is a limit to the taxation which is either tolerable by the people or compatible with a sound national economy. This truth is increasingly understood, but it is as true of health care as elsewhere. Acceptance of it must lead to belated acceptance of the principles upon which the system of financing health services outlined in our report was based.

XVII
A Strategy for Reform

John and Sylvia Jewkes

John Jewkes: *Professor of Social Economics, University of Manchester, 1936–46; Stanley Jevons Professor of Political Economy, University of Manchester, 1946–48; Professor of Economic Organisation and Fellow of Merton College, Oxford, 1948–69. Director of the Economic Section, War Cabinet Secretariat, 1941. Director General of Statistics and Programmes, Ministry of Aircraft Production, 1943. Member, Fuel Advisory Committee, 1945; Independent Member, Cotton Industry Working Party, 1946; Member, Royal Commission on Doctors' and Dentists' Remuneration, 1957–60.*

Sylvia Jewkes: *has collaborated with her husband in much of his writing. With him she co-authored "Juvenile Unemployment"; "The Genesis of the British National Health Service"; "Value for Money – in Medicine".*

How to reform the NHS so that it allows doctors to give patients the services they want? Some essays argue for fundamental reform sooner or later. In this essay Professor John and Mrs. Sylvia Jewkes, who courageously spoke out 20 or 25 years ago when critics of the NHS were condemned as almost immoral, here consider what reforms are practical that will conflict least sharply with [continuing] prejudices. They discuss tax refunds for private health insurance, incentives for family doctors, releasing the pressure on hospitals by homes financed by pension funds, and taking the teaching hospitals out of the NHS.

Introduction

It is always a mistake to abandon the search for the reform of some social or economic institution simply on the grounds that it is "politically impossible". Yet it is sensible to recognise that some reforms will be more difficult to carry out than others. With a fresh and determined government, the greater part of the vast tangle of controlling legislation which, since 1945, has pushed us towards a servile state might quickly be swept away. For it is becoming increasingly obvious that these controls are progressively restricting personal freedom and eroding economic incentives and few people have any good to say of them except legislators and bureaucrats who lovingly nurture and assiduously strive to extend them.

Prejudices obstructing reform

Sudden and radical changes in the NHS is another matter. This, even under the most favourable circumstances, will be the hardest nut to crack. Even Professor Hayek has written in *The Constitution of Liberty:*

> From what we have seen of such schemes (free health services for all) it is probable that their inexpediency will become evident in countries that have adopted them, although political circumstances make it unlikely that they can ever be abandoned.

So reforms will call for patience, step by step progress and the use of the thin end of the wedge. As has happened before, schemes for sweeping changes will quickly find themselves in pigeon holes.

This is a recognition of the almost pathological obsession on the part of the British public, in the face of all fact and logic, with the indestructible virtues of a comprehensive and free NHS. Even though the public is becoming increasingly aware of some defects (as, for instance, in the obvious cases where, now that at last a few new hospitals have been completed, they cannot be opened or fully used because there are no funds available) the only remedy envisaged is the allocation of more taxpayers' money to the NHS.

If British medical services are to be made more ample, efficient and progressive it will be in the teeth of opposition from many who would actually benefit from the change. It is, therefore, not a waste of time to plot the rocks which lie ahead.

NHS launched by myths

The NHS was launched with a series of mis-statements which, despite subsequent happenings, are dogmatically accepted. It was claimed that, before 1948, the existing medical services were poor and inferior to those in many other countries. This was untrue. The Service purports to provide free comprehensive medical services to everyone in need of them. This aim was clearly absurd since, with advance of medicine and the growing disinclination to tolerate minor physical ailments, the demand would be virtually without limit. But, far from foreseeing this likely outcome, the enthusiasts for the NHS argued that the annual expenditure would progressively make the nation healthier and automatically reduce costs. The cost rose from £180m in its first year to over £7,000m in 1978. Central government employment under the NHS rose from 575,000 in 1961 to 1,175,000 in 1978. And while, in 1961, NHS employment was about equal to that in H.M. Forces and the Police taken together, by

1978 the NHS was employing far more than twice as many.

The emotional grip which the idea of a free comprehensive health service has had on the public mind has produced unhappy consequences.

a) Whenever any useful commodity or service is offered free it is inescapable that the demand will outpace the supply. Some form of rationing has to be employed. In the NHS it has taken the form of waiting lists growing ever longer; medical and nursing staff being overworked and discouraged; and every government being accused of 'starving the Service'.

b) So long as the service offered is free (i.e. paid for out of general taxation) a low, even a falling standard of quality will be tolerated. This is remarkably true even with people who might be expected to notice and attach importance to any deterioration. Middle-class parents will, for instance, often courageously impoverish themselves to pay for a superior education for their children but are resigned to a free and inferior medical service for themselves and their families.

c) A free-for-all comprehensive health service lowers the standards of public morality. It generates hypocrisy and cynicism. It is well known that politicians who praise its so-called equality use private medical services and, even when they use the NHS, arrange for this to be widely reported (even though, because of their "importance", it is unlikely they will be called upon to take their place in the long queues). And, despite their obsessions with the sanctity of the NHS, there are trade union leaders, and trades unions, that subscribe to existing private medical insurance schemes.

"Equality" – a confidence trick

The so-called "equality" guaranteed by the NHS is a confidence trick. Since it is almost wholly paid for out of general taxation, it means that poorer people who are healthy and rarely go near a doctor may be meeting the costs of well-to-do people who are more frequently ill or disinclined to tolerate their minor afflictions.

The urge towards equality often turns into envy and masochism, and results in open declaration that it is preferable for every member of the community to suffer inferior medical services so long as no one has any advantage over another. Even so, the search for equality is a search for the impossible, since the capacity of doctors and the conditions under which they work vary enormously. In this sense the standard of treatment a patient receives will always be, in some measure, a matter of chance; but this, apparently, is not resented so long as everyone has the same chance in the lottery.

In the meantime many who bemoan the low level of medical services in developing countries (and urge that more British aid should be devoted to them) allow a situation to persist in which the NHS depends heavily on the services of many doctors from these poorer countries.

This passion for equality seems to deaden the power to link cause and effect. Thus the growth of private medical services which releases more resources for desirable public services is described as "queue-jumping" when, in the long run, it *shortens* the queue.

It is therefore not surprising that every Minister of Health since 1948, even those in Conservative governments who otherwise believed strongly in the virtues of the market economy, has found himself comparatively powerless when faced by this unique situation. It seems that no minister has thought it worthwhile to encourage, or even to take an active interest in the institutions providing insurance for private medical care. Some ministers have sought to explain away the defects of the NHS by pointing to the increase in the number of old people or the growing complexities of medical treatment. The last Labour government sought to put off the day of reckoning by appointing a Royal Commission on the NHS with terms of reference which barred it from discussing the question of pay beds, and therefore of private practice.

Breaking the vicious circle: reforms

If British medical services can be improved only by patient, piecemeal changes of a kind which will conflict least sharply with the prejudices and passions surrounding the subject, we advance the following suggestions.

The vicious circle which in some way has to be broken must clearly be recognised. A free service generates demand which first falls upon the general practitioner. His load becomes too heavy and he seeks to lighten it by passing cases on to the hospitals which, in turn, are swamped. The increasing total cost of the NHS, calling for increased taxation, leads government to try to restrict expenditure. One way of doing this is to try, by administrative devices, to control the activities of the medical profession, thus creating friction between the professionals and the administrators.

(i) *Taxation relief on private medical expenses*

A first general move would be to stimulate people to provide, to a higher degree than at present, for the costs of their medical services by allowing them to be deductible from taxable income. This is a practice, in varying forms, found in a number of countries.

These deductible costs might cover fees paid to the general practitioner for private service; charges met directly for hospital services: annual payments made to voluntary health schemes such as BUPA, payments made to insurance companies to cover possible future medical costs. The experience in other countries should provide guidance as to the relative benefits of the various measures of tax relief.

The two Founding Fathers of the NHS expected that, with the passage of time and growing prosperity, private medical services would increasingly supplement or take over from the public service. Aneurin Bevan, at the Labour Party Conference in 1945, said:

> If we were rich enough we would not want to have free medical services, we could pay the doctor.

Sir William Beveridge, in his famous Report "Social Insurance and Allied Services" published in 1942, recommended that:

> The State in organising security should not stifle incentive, opportunity, responsibility; in establishing a national minimum, it should leave room and encouragement for voluntary action by each individual to provide more than that minimum for himself and his family.

But although the real national income per head has at least doubled since 1945, and despite the personal examples set by the Founding Fathers (both in their later years made extensive use of private medical services) their hopes have been dashed. The monopoly of the NHS is still securely rivetted on the country.

We can only guess at the likely effect of this type of taxation relief: how many people would choose to opt out of state medical services and which services would be most affected. But it would be reasonable to hope for and expect some such consequences as these:

a) There would be a larger demand for private medical services of all kinds. Even if the changes were gradual there ought to be an increase in the number of private hospitals and increased entry into the medical profession. If the net effect was to raise the proportion of national income spent on all medical services in Britain to that in many other countries this could be regarded as highly encouraging.

b) We surmise that the British medical profession as a whole would not oppose this tax relief measure or that, if it did so, it would be on grounds which government might properly over-rule. Any increase in private medical services would most likely be to the advantage of those doctors and hospitals which enjoyed the highest reputation in the public mind. Some relief, therefore, from the present downward pressure on quality of service through the swamping of medical services might be expected. A further advantage might be that emigration would become less attractive and a return encouraged of some of the doctors who have left.

c) For the public generally the sense of personal responsibility and the satisfaction arising from the power to choose should be enhanced. In Britain the Family Expenditure Survey shows that only 0.2 per cent of total weekly household expenditure is devoted to "Medical Dental and Nursing Fees"; this is less than 3 per cent of the combined expenditure on alcohol and tobacco and about one half of net betting losses. British citizens take annually some 9 million holiday visits abroad; of British households 95 per cent own a television set; more than one half own one or more cars. It seems ridiculous to suppose that a significant slice of these households would not be prepared to economise on such luxuries if, thereby, they could be provided with improved amenities and refinements in medical services and were encouraged to do so by cutting the private cost through taxation relief.

The objection certain to be raised in some quarters would of course be that it would encourage "queue-jumping". In many fields the paranoic objection to "queue-jumping" has subsided with the disappearance of shortages, but it remains virulent in medical matters where the shortages continue to be the direct product of the NHS itself. Three answers might be given. First, the growth of private medical services would not necessarily weaken public medical services. Secondly, taxation relief does not free those who take advantage of it from their responsibility for continuing to pay taxes for the state medical service. It merely narrows the enormous gap between what the citizen gets free from the state service and what he pays for private service. Thirdly, it should not be supposed that, with a tax relief system, the better-off will necessarily opt out of the NHS more frequently than the rest. What would happen would depend upon the preferences, within the different income groups, for a better medical service as against competing amenities.

(ii) *Encourage family doctor*

The NHS has been something of a disaster for the family doctor. A flood of medical demand, much of it of trivial character, has been thrown upon him. Paperwork has multiplied, especially in claims for sickness benefits. All this in itself goes far to explain why doctors, as a simple defence, often send their patients to hospital and shift pressures one stage further on. Beyond this, whatever may have been the professional pride and integrity of the family doctor, his incentives have been weakened by the manner in which he is paid. The capitation fee system provides no reward, except personal satisfaction, for care and effort. In any case the capitation fee is so derisory that the practitioner is tempted to take on a maximum list in order to make a living.

This cuts down the time he has available for each patient. (The Secretary of the British Medical Association has quite properly complained of the low capitation fee. But he then went on to say that this, in itself, would drive more practitioners into the private sector and 'this would be tragic'. Is it the accepted policy of the BMA to discourage private practice?) Would the introduction of some form of "fee for service" not help here? The GP might be left to choose between "capitation fee" and "fee for item of service". Additional administrative complications might be created by such an option. But to continue to pay all doctors with the same size list the same income, where variations in skill and application differ enormously, would seem to invite slackness and dissatisfaction.

It seems certain that private general practice has fallen off rapidly in recent years. It would certainly be encouraged by the abolition of the rule, often attacked but staunchly defended by every Government since 1948, that anyone who chose to pay for the services of the general practitioner is, thereby, debarred from obtaining his prescribed medicines free, or heavily subsidised, from the NHS. This is a bureaucratic rule which is resented by many practitioners who believe that a measure of private practice is conducive to efficiency and enthusiasm in their work.

(iii) *Release the pressure on the hospitals*

The overcrowding in the hospitals and the lengthening of waiting lists may, to some degree, be relieved by these measures. But it will remain serious for a long time unless some drastic decisions are made fairly promptly. About one half of all hospital beds are occupied by old people. Some are properly there as needing medical treatment of an advanced kind but many are simply needing agreeable accommodation with more economical but nevertheless quite adequate and kindly care, far short of the medical services for which hospitals should cater.

The usual solution to this dilemma in British minds is for the State to take on still heavier burdens by building old peoples' homes. But here private effort should be fully evoked. One obvious step would be for Occupational Pension Funds to provide the means for creating and maintaining accommodation for their pensioners who need and desire it. Some Pension Funds, particularly of the nationalised industries, have reached gigantic proportions: the National Coal Board Fund now exceeds £2,000m. And, if the report is correct, they do not always find it easy to invest their assets to advantage. To provide suitable homes for their pensioners who opt for them would be an imaginative act, at once catering in a sympathetic and intimate way for their own pensioners and reducing the burden of tax on the general public.

(iv) *Extract the Teaching Hospitals from the NHS*

People obsessed with the case for equality will be driven to endanger new and established centres of excellence. The great British teaching hospitals, with their outstanding reputation for research and advances in the higher levels of treatment have, to that extent, always been in danger since 1948. The danger has proved real and the teaching hospitals have been pushed continually towards supplying general community services rather than developing as centres for research and training. The danger grows. Some Ministers of Health have, in the name of equality, engaged themselves in what can only properly be described as social vandalism, by enforcing cuts in the budgets of London's most famous teaching hospitals, so weakening their teaching roles. With a new Conservative government, in order to settle this matter once and for all, serious consideration should be given to taking the teaching hospitals out of the National Health Service altogether and, in effect, making them a part of the University system.

The funds for the teaching hospitals might be channelled through the University Grants Committee (already many doctors in these hospitals are paid by the Universities) and the Boards of Governors be resurrected. This reform would go as far as possible in rendering the teaching hospitals free from political control. They should be encouraged, as indeed all hospitals should be encouraged, to raise outside funds. If the public were to be made fully aware of the enormous cost of the various treatments provided "free" it might be more inclined to contribute generously.

And, since we all value most what we pay for, it would help to sweep away, after 32 years, the most bizarre socialist dream that has ever bedevilled our people; the illusion that the State can provide all and every medical service and medicament to every man, woman and child, native and foreign, without discouraging economy, creating shortages and debasing quality.

XVIII

Better Medicine by Better Insurance

Hugh Elwell

Born 1932. Educated Newport Grammar School. Joined Army from school. Left in 1957 to join the British United Provident Association (BUPA) as Management Trainee. Left in 1976 as **General Manager and member of the Board.** *Has travelled widely and lectured extensively in the USA on health care in the UK. Has observed at first hand the American health services. Adviser to Private Patients Plan (PPP).*

If more people want to escape from the NHS, how will they pay for the alternative – by fees for family doctors, consultants and hospitals. The larger fees, especially for hospitals, are reduced to manageable sums by health insurance. In this essay Hugh Elwell, with over 20 years practical experience, discusses likely developments in health insurance as it expands and diversifies its services to meet growing public demand. He envisages new insurers appearing to provide new schemes in competition with the existing provident funds.

Introduction

Health insurance – or more aptly, ill-health insurance – in the United Kingdom is still in its infancy. A comprehensive NHS, mainly tax funded and to all intents and purposes "free" at point of consumption, has discouraged initiatives by insurance companies to provide cover against the cost of private medical treatment.

Of the companies in the field, two are profit-making but account for only 1 per cent of the total market share. Of the remainder, three non-profit funds cover about 98 per cent of the total market. These, the Provident Associations, have been the organisations to which anyone requiring data about health insurance has turned, not because they are necessarily the best source of information but because they are the only source. To a large extent, therefore, discussion about the relevance of insurance in paying for medical treatment has centred around the experience of the major Provident Associations. Their benefits are based on the principles of "pecuniary loss" – a claim is paid only for the amount of money expended. And the initiatives in health insurance have inevitably been coloured by the view that so far the market for this type of cover has been strictly limited. After thirty years of the NHS the number of persons covered by health insurance is still only about 2.5 million out of 55 million.

From individual (family) to group (employee) insurance cover

Some changes in the subscriber population of the major Provident Associations, however, have substantial implications that have been so far inadequately thought through by them. But they have considerable relevance in the discussion about the wider role of health insurance.

In the days immediately following the introduction of the NHS the Associations providing health insurance dealt almost exclusively with the individual as an individual risk, with premium based solely on the claims experience of all individuals covered within defined age groups. In the main, the benefits provided a given sum of money for the cost of a defined item of service, whether per day in hospital or for a consultant's procedure.

This system of rating of premiums has been increasingly changed for some sections of the insured population as the concept of the group coverage has been developed. Here, the company buys for a range of its employees a block of insurance cover, with the guarantee that there is no selection against the insurer – all eligible employees are covered. This method thus reduces the individual risk to the insurer, and obtains for the company a reduced insurance rate (average "community" as opposed to individual "experience" rating).

An extension to this development has been what amounts increasingly to virtually open-ended benefits, with maximum limits unlikely to be exceeded by any of the insured.

It must be stressed, however, that after some unsatisfactory experience with providing cover for general practitioner services, the Provident Associations now supply insurance only for consultants, in their private rooms or in hospitals, and for hospital services.

More emphasis on cost control

The implications of this change of emphasis are considerable. The item-of-service

110

element that was and still is of great importance in the make-up of the individual's insurance cover has largely disappeared in the company coverage. But the necessity to establish some form of cost control with the suppliers of private treatment has been so far inadequately pursued. With only a very small percentage population insured, it would be of little importance.

It assumes more relevance, however, when it is seen increasingly that employers, and indeed now trade unions, are seeking coverage for substantial segments of the workforce. Total insurance coverage for all consultant service "episodes" can lead to a dramatic rise in both claims rate and premiums. In essence, no price control over demand could lead to over utilisation, and ultimately some form of benefit "rationing".

New competition

Another, and possibly more significant, result of an increasing demand by the workforce for health insurance is the certainty of new insurers entering what has historically been the province of the non-profit insurance associations (with the two minor exceptions). Hitherto, the major commercial insurance groups have paid little attention to what has always been considered a minor field of activity and one, futhermore, that has always attracted a degree of political opprobrium from one major political party and little but vague support from the other.

As it now stands, the market for health insurance could cover at least four times the present insured population, or about 10 million. With the continuing deterioration of the NHS and its ability to supply a service at the time and place to suit the patient, this market will develop dramatically, in particular when new and consumer-oriented insurers enter the field. Virile competition will stimulate the existing funds into re-thinking the range of their product.

It will also have the effect of demonstrating that, even with the necessary provisos of the Department of Trade requirements for a stable fund, insurance is capable of an almost infinite variety of coverage, depending on the requirements of any part of the population at any time. As competition increases, insurance will be geared to the demands of different sectors of the market. To the traditional system of indemnity insurance will be added co-insurance – where the insured person pays a given proportion of the cost of the service received, and a deductible system – where the insured pays a given initial sum before the insurance cover takes over. In the major (particularly multi-national) companies, there will certainly be a move towards self-insurance, where the company itself covers its own insurance risks, possibly from an offshore fund.

Extension of coverage

The next few years will see a dramatic increase in both the numbers of people insured against the cost of private medical treatment, and in the number of the providers of insurance. Similarly, the types of cover available will develop to suit both the growing market and the changing pattern of care available. And the competition that develops will provide the necessary incentive for the insurance companies to seek a balance between maximum benefits and minimum premiums.

The effectiveness with which a correct balance is established will depend largely on the ability of the insurers to develop to the full cost-control arrangements with both the insured population and with hospitals' consultants, family doctors and other suppliers of health services. Over-utilisation of the insurance fund benefits would lead to an escalation of premiums, as it does where there is no control by competition over the charges made by the medical profession and by the suppliers of hospital beds. Recognition by the insured population will quickly be given when it is seen that those insurance funds that are the most effective in controlling costs are able to charge lower premiums for their cover than are charged by their competitors who do not attempt to control costs.

So far, I have discussed broadly the development of health insurance since the inception of the NHS and the likely trend over the next few years. In the longer term, it is perfectly feasible to imagine the NHS becoming at least in part, if not fully, funded by insurance, rather than by taxes.

The two inherent problems of any insurance-based activity, moral hazard and adverse selection, could be readily overcome by the appropriate benefit structure, and by the development of experience rating. The impact of the moral hazard on an insurance scheme is a change in the pattern of behaviour of the person covered. A non-insurance illustration is the misuse of a GP's time by a patient with a trivial complaint who would never have considered going to the doctor had the service not been "free". The problem of adverse selection is one where a high-risk person tends to buy, or buy more, insurance than a low-risk person. The larger the proportion of the high-risk insured persons in a given insurance pool, the more the likelihood of a high claims rate – leading to the inevitability of increased premiums. With complete coverage of a given population, whether a company's staff or a complete community, selection against the insurer is removed, with the result of lower premiums.

The public and health insurance

The attitude of the general public towards the NHS as a "cradle to the grave" provider of medical care has been surprisingly little disturbed by the muted promotion of ill-health insurance by the Provident Association. Research by two of them suggests that there is still a relatively high degree of satisfaction with the "free" NHS. At the same time, it is apparent that there is a growing awareness of the existence of ill-health insurance; awareness, but not necessarily a likelihood to buy. This is understandable since most people have no idea what the NHS cost is to them. A popular misconception is that an element of the National Insurance contribution pays for the whole of the NHS. Little wonder, therefore, if the individual who sends off for details of health insurance finds the premium cost far in excess of what he anticipated since he had, hitherto, no means of knowing what he was already contributing to the NHS, and no means of valuing in money terms the health care he received.

The lack of public education on the real cost of the NHS is one of the major tasks in the development of ill-health insurance. The existing insurers could do more than they do. But until the commercial insurers enter the field by offering ill-health insurance as a normal part of the "household all-risks" policy, the average family will have little idea of the relative cost of ill-health insurance against that of car or fire insurance.

A question of facilities

A dramatic rise in the number of people seeking private medical care would clearly present a problem for the suppliers. Those facilities that would create the biggest "bottleneck" in the short term are the "bricks and mortar": the hospitals, operating theatres, etc.: medical manpower would be far more elastic in meeting new demand. The flexibility of the private sector would ensure that far more use was made of existing trained nursing staff who, because they can work only part-time, are under-used by the NHS.

Although it takes a minimum of two years to create a new private hospital, the time element is not the most crucial; undoubtedly the main problem is cost. Capital for new hospital projects is readily available. A number of profit-making hospitals are being, or have been, built, but at a cost in excess of charitable hospitals, where there is normally no capital to service. An escalation of "for profit" hospitals will inevitably lead to higher bed charges, which in turn will be reflected in premium rates. Yet there will certainly be a demand for the minimum amount of time to be spent in hospital in post-operative care. The patient would be sent home at the earliest possible opportunity. This would place both a burden and an opportunity on the family doctor who, at present, sees no benefit in the development of private medicine or an increase in the number of private patients; but it would reduce the claim on the insurance fund.

XIX

The NHS as a Nationalised Industry

Alfred Sherman

Journalist, writer, economic and public affairs adviser. Director of Studies and co-founder of the Centre for Policy Studies. Writings include: "Tito, a Reluctant Revisionist"; "Capitalism and Freedom"; "The Chinese Peoples' Communes"; "The years of the Left Book Club"; "The Complacent Satirists".

Hugh Elwell argued that much or most of the NHS could be financed by insurance (although some "public" health services would remain to be financed by rates or taxes). He is followed by two essayists who argue for the radical approach of de-nationalisation. Alfred Sherman briefly outlines the general case against the nationalisation of medical care.

Introduction

Socialism and other secular religions owe some of their success to sustained misuse of words. One term which has misled many is "social services". We are told that social services are a good thing, should be supplied by the state, and are (or should be) above economics. 'Housing is (or should be) a social service', the propagandists declaim, thereby obviating economic (or any other) analysis.

I contend that there is no such thing as a "social service". It is simply a term used to describe any *private* services or goods (as distinct from "public goods" proper which must be supplied by government because they must be financed by taxes) because at any given time they happen to be distributed free, or at below cost at point of consumption, by the state, or because someone thinks they should be so distributed. Medicine and education are thus wrongly classed as "social services"; legal services and other professional services less so, though there is some creeping socialism there too.

In Britain, food is not regarded as a social service, except in the growing custom of ascribing to the state the duty of feeding children.

State feeding was originally advocated on the grounds that school meals were a convenience. They are now demanded on the grounds that many working-class parents cannot be relied on to feed their children, therefore the state should feed all. In countries where food production and distribution is treated like a social service – the Communist world and some third-world Marxified states like Tanzania – the people half-starve, and would do so completely were it not for generous Western food supplied at below cost.

Health services are a nationalised industry

It follows that health provision and state education must be treated conceptually in the same way as British Leyland, the National Coal Boad, Post Office and other nationalised industries. Differences can be found between every one of them and its fellows. Some hold monopolies and some are forced to compete. Of these, some offer a free or subsidised service at the point of use against full-cost private provision – and often lose the competition. Health education and shipbuilding are in the first category: ship-repairing and BL in the second. Some were initiated from the outset as outdoor relief for highly-unionised staff – mining, shipbuilding, BL. Others were designed initially to serve the consumer – health and education. But all have tended to assimilate to a single pattern in time.

They increasingly serve the immediate interests of the staff, irrespective of the public interests or the long-term interests of the service. They downgrade their supply of information to a point where it becomes increasingly difficult to test the relative efficiency of their various parts. They press for monopoly powers in order to outlaw the competition which exposes their inefficiency. Their short-sighted egoism is dressed up in idealistic language.

The NHS was begun by socialist doctrinaires without any clear idea of the problem of health service or of underlying concepts. No one has adequately defined "health service". I personally question whether it is amenable to definition, let alone measurement. One can, with certain caveats, measure the health of the population, over time and even with cautious inter-state comparisons. But what part of this should be ascribed to health service provision, as distinct from public health, diet, and so on?

No one has been able to do this so far.

And where does health provision end and personal comfort begin?

Rational management impossible

Without criteria, no rational management or measurement is possible. So the main pressures are for increasing expenditures in default of other and more rigorous guidelines. The pressures come increasingly from inside for a number of reasons.

Members of decision-making and opinion-forming circles are least likely to suffer from the inadequacies of the NHS. Most enjoy either privileged facilities from the state or access to non-state facilities. This is true of a high proportion of trade union officials, Labour MPs, left-wing journalists. And it is true of what have come to be described as paternalistic Tories – though their concept of paternalism might best be called Edomite, since it entails the sacrifice of others' children to false gods: comprehensives, child-centred education, etc. They have no concern other than to win political good will. This is most easily done by giving the state other people's money and leaving its institutions to work out for themselves how they will spend it.

Cuts and restraint are made difficult by bureaucrat and trade union control, which offloads all cuts onto the most deserving and politically sensitive services, leaving bureaucracy, waste and overmanning untouched.

Demoralisation affects all classes equally. To put it another way, all classes are proletarianised. The white-collar staff soon pick up the trade unionist combination of utter selfishness and high-flown jargon. (Few would rely on the benevolence of trade union leaders for their treatment.)

Worse still, professions like medicine are in danger of losing the essence of their professionalism, which lies in a direct relationship with the client, as they become salaried employees.

These considerations make nonesense of repeated claims that the NHS can be reformed, any more than any other nationalised industry can. The consumer market-disciplines which make for efficiency are not there, and cannot be introduced without dismantling the system. This change will be brought about from the top, or from the bottom as the union members' self interest clashes with their masters' ideology and family health with trade union solidarity, so that they themselves demand health insurance from employers.

XX
De-Nationalise NHS by Private Health Insurance

Andrew Moncreiff

Early life in Rhodesia; studied engineering at Cambridge; after a time in the construction industry moved to stockbroking and then to financial planning, initially running own business, subsequently with a merchant bank. Now investment manager for a forestry management company.

The case against nationalising medical care has been argued in principle in previous essays. Here Andrew Moncreiff attempts a detailed calculation of the tax costs of the NHS and the insurance costs of private health services.

Introduction

When discussing the provision of health care it is nearly always necessary to counter two myths which appear to be almost indelibly imprinted on the public consciousness:

> "The National Health Service is cheap and excellent value for money"

and

> "Private Insurance is prohibitively expensive for all but the super-rich"

The truth is that in 1979 the NHS cost £8,535 million and an increase of 17% would raise the cost for the current year to £10,000 million or £179 per head of population. thus a family of four is paying over £700 a year to support the NHS – £13.76 a week – and that covers only the running costs. The same family of four would pay less than a third of this to obtain private health insurance cover although the range of services is of course different. (A leading health insurance group would cover a family for £186 a year if both parents are under 30, or £206.64 if either is aged 30 or over. In practice nearly all subscribers can obtain a discount of at least 10% off these published scales.)

This essay attempts to find a basis for a valid comparison.

A comparison of state and market costs

As a starting point it is necessary to derive an average private insurance premium for an actuarially typical population. This can be done by considering two cases of a child born into a typical two-child family, growing up to marry and support two children, and dying at the actuarially expected age of 70 (male) and 76 (female). The premiums are those quoted by a leading health insurance group for a scale of benefits which covers the costs of more than 80% of the country's hospitals. It is assumed that the bread-winner is a member of a large company insurance scheme in which a discount of 40% is obtained against the published scales (this discount appears to be in line with current practice). For these actuarial models of typical lives the average premium per individual per year is £50.18.

Various adjustments must then be made.

Private insurance does not cover general medical, dental, ophthalmic or drugs expenditure, which account for about 24% of NHS costs. Scaling the private premium up in this proportion to include these services indicates that a premium of £66 per head would be required.

The private group from which these figures were drawn was able to set 25% of its income aside last year either for capital expenditure or to reserves (the previous year it was almost 30%). The NHS costs, quoted above, contain no provision for reserves or for capital expenditure and to get a strict comparison the private sector premium should be reduced by 25%. In practice however we would always expect some provision for reserves in a privately funded system, probably of the order of 10% of income, and on this premise the private premium is reduced by 15%, to £56.

The private cover contains certain exclusions which limit liability and these fall into two categories:–

(i) Geriatric

14½% of the population are over 65. In the actuarial model of a privately insured population 25% of the premiums are paid by people over 65 but they account for 36% of the costs of the NHS. Part of the cost of geriatric care in the NHS is really "welfare" rather than medical because of the failure of other branches of the welfare system, but nevertheless, increasing the premiums of those over 65 in the private model to the full 36% of the total gives a new average individual premium of £66.

(ii) *Medical catastrophe*

Many critics of private health care have claimed that medical catastrophe is uninsurable but, on the contrary, it is a classic example of an insurable risk since the cost is beyond the means of all but a few individuals but the risk can be covered for a very small premium over a large population because of the rare occurrence of the disaster. However, for the same reason that an individual must insure against a risk of this type, an insurer covering a small 'self-selected' population cannot carry that risk. It is largely for this reason that the medical insurers have chosen to limit their liability. It is interesting to note here that this policy has also resulted in a limitation of their facilities since they have had no incentive to acquire the equipment necessary to treat medical catastrophe although the capital is available for its provision.

Over a large population the cost of medical catastrophe is small and as the insured population approaches the total population the risk can be calculated and financed. With the exception of geriatric care (considered above) the exclusions have recently been substantially reduced without any increase in premium levels and most large company schemes now being negotiated have no limits at all. The remaining limits and exclusions could probably be removed without a significant change in financial terms but to be conservative an increase of 10% is assumed here, adding a further 10% to the average private insurance premium to £72.35.

We have now arrived at a notional cost *per capita* of providing complete and comprehensive private health insurance cover for a large, actuarially typical group based on current rates and costs and current medical practice. This figure of £72.35 is well under half the £179 per head which is the current cost of running the NHS.

Other influences on private health costs

About three-quarters of the cost of the NHS is absorbed by the hospital service and there can be little doubt that private insurers could make considerable savings compared with the rates now built into their premium scales. In order to compete with a "free" service the private sector sells privacy, colour television, a more personal service etc. and it charges accordingly. In an open market the rich would still pay extra for their privacy and convenience but the general service could be very significantly cheaper. A simple awareness of economics should lead to further savings through, for example, greater use of para-medical facilities particularly nursing and convalescent homes, protected housing for the elderly, or cash subsidies for those convalescents able to make their own arrangements in the local community or in their own family.

On the other hand the private sector would have to upgrade their existing facilities. To the extent that these facilities already exist in the NHS they would presumably be available (by hire or transfer) to the private sector if the bulk of the population wished to be cared for privately. To the extent that new capital is required the money will have to be provided by the people of Britain one way or another in any event. It makes little difference to a comparative study such as this whether they do so through taxes or insurance premiums, or, indeed, charitable donations.

The private sector could probably not run family doctoring more cheaply than the state because in a private service the GP would find himself spending more time with each patient and making more home visits. The service would be better and no doubt most GPs would welcome the opportunity to provide this better service, but it would be more expensive than the present "utility" NHS service. Some of this extra cost would, however, be recovered through an easing of pressure on the hospitals particularly the casualty wards.

The price of drugs might increase with the decline in the monopoly purchasing power of the state but a better and more personal service from GPs might lead to a compensating fall in the volume of drugs prescribed.

These influences pull in different directions but taken together they should reduce health care costs. They cannot be quantified in advance and no allowance is made for them here.

Public opinion and future policy

A recent investigation for the Institute of Economic Affairs indicated that 78% of the population were in favour of arrangements to contract out of the NHS as a general principle. More specifically, just over half said that they themselves would contract out if the government offered a voucher of half the cost of private insurance.

Suppose the government were to take existing pension arrangements as a precedent and allow people to contract out of the nationalised health service, rebating half of the cost of private insurance through Income Tax, Corporation Tax or National Insurance contributions. On the evidence of the I.E.A. survey, mentioned above, we would expect a majority to contract out and this majority would probably grow as the idea became more familiar, limited primarily by the ability of the private sector to provide facilities, both medical and administrative.

The trend towards company health insurance schemes would probably continue and consolidate with the impetus coming as much from the unions as from employers once the trend was firmly established. It is worth noting that in South Africa where private health insurance is almost universal among whites, well over 95% are covered through company schemes. Many companies allow outsiders to join, thus allowing the self-employed and employees without a company scheme to benefit from their low premiums.

For the small minority not in a company scheme and with insufficient income to claim the full reliefs other arrangements would have to be made (e.g. direct subsidies as in the "Option Mortgage" scheme). It is important to stress that this lack of purchasing power is not a problem in the supply of health care and has nothing to tell us about the relative merits of different systems of health care delivery. It is a "welfare" problem to do with income maintenance or the relief of poverty in general.

Financial effects of contracting out

Suppose, after the transitional period, (a) 50% and (b) 80% of the population had contracted out.

(a) With 50% contracted out the cost of the tax relief would be £1,010 million at 1980 prices, leaving £8,990 million, or 90% of its present funding, available to the NHS to provide for the remaining half of the population. By hiring surplus facilities to the private sector the NHS might even be able to maintain the finance available to it.

(b) With 80% contracted out the tax-relief would be £1,620 million, leaving the NHS with £8,380 million, or 84% of its present resources, to provide for 20% of the population. If the Treasury were to take £2,500 million annually to reduce the budget deficit the NHS would have three-fifths of its present budget to care for one fifth of the population.

The transitional period

The transition would raise many issues and problems outside the scope of a purely financial analysis.

The worst possible financial effects would occur if 50% of the population were contracted out and claiming tax-relief before any savings were seen in the NHS and without any increase in private (fee-paying) use of NHS facilities. The cost to the Exchequer would then be £1,010 million on an annual basis. Even this hypothetical worst case might be an acceptable policy option since it implies a huge improvement in the standard of health care which could not be achieved as cheaply any other way.

If the numbers contracting out rose to 50% over four years and the first savings in the NHS were seen only in the third year (2%, rising to 4% in the fourth year), but one fifth of the additional private expenditure returned to the NHS through the hire or purchase of NHS facilities or staff time, then the net loss to the Exchequer might be £160 million in the first year, £260 million in the second, £210 million in the third year and £150 million in the fourth. The savings in the NHS would have to reach 6½% in the fifth year to achieve a break-even position.

There has been much discussion about the best uses to which the North Sea Oil revenues should be put. Surely anyone's shortlist should include the temporary cost of reorganising our health care in such a way as to yield financial benefits in the long term, an increase in individual liberty and, not least, better health care for all. More important perhaps, is that if we do not take this opportunity very soon it is almost certain that very much larger sums will have to be spent on saving the NHS from total collapse.

XXI
"The Envy of the World"?

John Goodman

*Assistant Professor of Economics at the University of Dallas, Texas,
Co-author of "Economics of Public Policy" and author of two
forthcoming books: "National Health Care in Great Britain:
Lessons for the U.S."; and "Social Security: The British Experience".*

*We are in no doubt that the NHS must be radically reformed or
replaced. But do other countries see more to admire? Where have
they copied, or adapted it? Nowhere except in the Communist
world. What of the Western world? Professor John Goodman from
the USA, where living standards are twice as high as in Britain,
but whose medical services have been strongly condemned in
Britain, claims his country provides better services. He presents a
very different state of affairs from the one made familiar by British
critics. American services concentrate on curing; British services
use resources for "caring" with little effect on health. British
curing services would be considered "shockingly inadequate" in
the USA. Professor Goodman illustrates his argument from the
emergency care of ambulances, primary (family doctor) services (no
regular check-ups in the NHS), preventive medicine (less in the
UK), hospital services for "acute" patients, the much higher
percentage of specialists in the USA, the much lower frequency of
visits to family doctors in the USA, quality of buildings, quality of
doctors, expenditure on modern technology (renal dialysis), and
other services.*

1. U.S.A.: HEALTH SERVICES ARE SUPERIOR

Introduction

'Put people before buildings.' That was the way a 1976 Consultative Document summarised the philosophy behind its recommended spending priorities for the NHS budget. That philosophy embodied two distinct preferences: (1) a desire to give more priority to current over capital expenditure, and (2) a desire to give more priority to routine and less expensive treatment over newer, more expensive and more potent techniques.

The clear winners in the proposed budget changes were the chronically ill, the elderly and the handicapped. The clear losers were the acutely ill. The Consultative Document showed a marked preference for the "caring" over the "curing" functions of health care. Medical techniques which can save lives and cure diseases were to take a back seat to those which merely increase the comfort of patients.

"Curing" more important than "caring"

To me as an American observer of the NHS, this philosophy is difficult to understand. For the biggest difference between the two is not that the American is basically private while British medicine is basically public. Nor is it that Americans spend two to three times as much *per capita* on medical care as the British do. It is the difference in spending priorities.

Even before the Consultative Document's proposals began to take effect, the NHS was spending far more of its budget on "caring" and much less on "curing" than in the United States. The NHS provides millions of non-acute patients with medical services that are virtually non-existent on this side of the Atlantic. These services only marginally affect health, and perhaps not at all. On the other hand, the care provided by the NHS to the acutely ill would be considered shockingly inadequate – even verging on the inhumane – in the USA.

I illustrate this fundamental contrast from recent British and American writings and reports. (The full documentation is in my book *National Health Care in Great Britain*, 1980.

Emergency care

In 1976, there were 21.7 million ambulance journeys in England; almost one for every two people. Yet only 1.5 million were for genuine medical emergencies. Over 93 per cent were described in the Merrison Report as little more than a free "taxi service".

When a real emergency (such as a heart attack or stroke) does occur, the ambulance service is poorly equipped to deal with it. NHS ambulances rarely contain a paramedic or an emergency medical technician (EMT). Very few ambulances have radio links or sophisticated emergency care equipment. Not only is the ambulance service notoriously slow in responding to real medical emergencies; whole areas of South East England, South Wales and Scotland are largely without any emergency facilities.

In the United States, ambulances are almost exclusively reserved for medical emergencies. Moreover, in most large American cities ambulances generally carry paramedics or EMTs and have radio links with hospital doctors. Far from being a surrogate taxi, the typical American ambulance is a mobile emergency treatment centre.

Primary care

Most Americans are amazed to learn that British general practitioners make house calls. Even if the visits are often made by "deputy doctors", the service sounds attractive to citizens of a country where home visits are almost extinct. I would guess that British GPs may make as many as 1.75 million house calls annually at a total cost to the NHS of perhaps £30m. Yet for the kinds of service most American patients expect from their family doctor, British general practitioner service is woefully inadequate. In the USA people are generally encouraged to get an annual physical examination, called a "check-up" – blood tests, a urine test, a chest X-ray, etc., usually in the general practitioner's office. It is similar to that offered by the BUPA Medical Centre in London. Within the NHS, however, the general "check-up" is virtually unknown.

This is not surpising. In contrast with their American counterparts, most British GPs have few instruments beyond a stethoscope and blood pressure cuffs and often must send their patient to the hospital for chest X-rays and simple blood tests. Even if the British GP were able to offer more extensive services he does not have the time; on the average less than five minutes per patient compared with 12 to 13 minutes in the USA.

Far less preventive medicine is practised in Britain than in the USA. Despite the high hopes of Aneurin Bevan that the NHS would encourage preventive treatment when health care was made free at the point of consumption, it is strikingly rare by American standards. Only 8 per cent of all eligible women in Britain receive an annual PAP smear. Even the Merrison Report expressed alarm at the low vaccination rate for every major childhood disease.

Dr Nicholas Krikes, President of the California Medical Association, said after a visit to England: 'In this town of Wycombe – with no appreciable slums, excellent light industry and in general a very beautiful town – there were 245 cases of measles last year. If we had 245 cases of measles in my city, which has three times the population, there would be considerable consternation and corrective effort.

The British record on preventive medicine may be partly due to a difference in attitude between British and American patients. The more fundamental reason, as with the ambulance service, relates to NHS priorities. Although the NHS may spend as much as £30m on house calls, it refuses to furnish GPs with the equipment most American doctors have, and gives GPs weak financial incentives to purchase equipment on their own. GPs also have weak financial incentives to offer many of the preventive services they are capable of performing. British doctors, for example, rarely give their female patients PAP smears or breast checks unless the patients insist on the treatment.

Hospital care

An American perspective on the British hospital sector was vividly summarised by economist, Mary-Ann Rozbicki, after a visit to a new hospital in York. She found that it compared very favourably with American hospitals for services rendered to *non*-acute patients. The hospital featured a complete gymnasium with a full-time therapist, a hydrotherapy unit with pool and mechanical lifting/dipping device; a job-oriented industrial machine unit; handicrafts and other occupational therapy equipment; and a complete kitchen for self-help orientation. Yet although the hospital contained a coronary care unit, there was *not one cardiological specialist on the hospital staff.*

Nor is this example unique. Rozbicki writes: 'In the East Anglian Region, 1974 data show that, of the 2.67 acute beds available per 1000 population, only 0.02 were earmarked for cardiology (the same as for dermatology and less than for plastic surgery). Moreover, the number was that high only because of the availability in Cambridge District hospitals; no beds were earmarked for cardiological patients in the entire Norfolk and Suffolk areas nor in the Peterborough District of Cambridge-shire'. Heart disease, incidentally, is the second leading cause of days of incapacity and the leading cause of death in Britain.

Statistics such as these are difficult for Americans to understand. Equally perplexing is that while large numbers of patients with life-threatening conditions cannot gain immediate entrance into British hospitals, many beds earmarked for acute care are filled with patients whose presence in the hospital is medically unnecessary. In 1977 there were 40,000 "urgent" patients on hospital waiting lists, while 25 per cent of all *acute* beds were occupied by *chronic* patients who theoretically should not have been there at all.

Caring versus curing

The most dramatic contrasts between the caring and curing functions of the NHS occurs between branches of the NHS. Take the contrast between general practitioner services and the services of specialists. About 17 per cent of all American physicians are general practitioners. In Britain, the percentage is about three times as high. In the USA the average patient sees his GP about *once* every year, compared with *four* visits in Britain. In both countries the majority of GP visits are for conditions which are medically trivial: the GP does little more than offer comfort and reassurance. But Britain is clearly devoting much more of its resources to this kind of care. In return, British patients pay a price: widespread shortages of specialists throughout the country. Many surgical specialities are found only in regional or teaching hospitals. Patients often have to travel a considerable distance for relatively unsophisticated treatment – provided they can travel and can gain admission.

Community services

Or take the contrast between the community health sector and the hospital sector. In 1976, nearly 8 million house calls were made by home nurses and health visitors in Great Britain: the equivalent of 14 per cent of the British population and perhaps one-half of all British households. In addition, over 1.3 million visits were made to patients' homes by chiropodists. About 172,000 people were served in their homes by the "meals on wheels" programme, and approximately 653,000 elderly and handi-capped people received "home help service" for house alterations, personal applicances (telephones, televisions and radios), and other arrangements that permit them to live at home. In the United States, there is some home visiting by nurses and there are a few "meals on wheels" programmes. but the number of these home visits *per capita* in the USA is a tiny fraction of that in Britain.

Hospital services

If community health services seem lavish by American standards, hospital services seem skimpy. Over 700,000 people are now waiting to enter British hospitals (over 40,000 classified as "urgent"). The British press and medical journals are filled with horror stories of patients dying because they were not properly admitted and treated. Moreover, many of the "non-urgent" cases wait for years in constant pain; many others wait at considerable personal risk. In the Liverpool-Wellington area, for example, children in need of hole-in-the-heart operations face a two-year to three-year wait – which doctors believe may jeopardise their chances of survival.

Yet there are fewer hospital beds in Britain today than there were when the NHS was started. Moreover, the hospitals that house them are often outmoded, ill-equipped and understaffed. Over 50 per cent of all beds are in buildings built before the turn of the century. These buildings Professor Michael Cooper has described as 'obsolete' and 'offering facilities in many respects more akin to a railway station than a place for the ailing'.

Quality of doctors

If the NHS has failed to maintain the quality of its buildings, it has done little more to maintain the quality of its medical staff. Britain is losing many of its best doctors to foreign countries and to the private sector. The annual number of emigrant doctors equals about 15 per cent of each year's graduating class from British medical schools. About 66 per cent of all hospital consultants have a private practice and work only part time for the NHS. These doctors have been replaced by immigrant doctors from countries like India and Nigeria. About 30 per cent of all hospital doctors are foreign born. Yet while British doctors are well-trained, there is considerable doubt about the quality of their replacements. When a qualifying test was administered to foreign-born doctors during the first six months of 1975, two-thirds failed the exam.

As for the quality of other services rendered in the NHS hospitals, consider the following: in 1970, *27 per cent of all known cases of food poisoning in Britain occurred in hospitals* – more than all of the cases occurring in restaurants, clubs and canteens combined. In that same year, the USA Centre for Disease Control reported *not a single case* of food poisoning in a USA hospital.

Equally startling to Americans is the contrast between the amount of money spent on family practitioner services and on modern medical technology. In 1976, the NHS spent over £47.3m subsiding dentures. It spent over £24m giving people "free" eyesight tests. In 1975 it spent almost £4.5m subsidising contraceptives and millions more on "free" contraceptive counselling.

Yet in 1975 and 1976 up to 7560 people may have died in Britain because the NHS refused to provide them with renal dialysis. The decision, in 1978, to purchase 400 additional dialysis units will put only a small dent in this number. In the USA there are very few government subsidies for dentures, eyesight tests, or contraceptive devices, but it is doubtful that any American patient dies because he is denied access to renal dialysis.

In 1975, the NHS spent over £6m on sleeping pills, almost £8.9m on tranquilisers and sedatives, £5.5m on cough medicine, almost £2m on vitamins and millions more on bandaids, cotton wool and items of comparable medical importance. These numbers appear especially incredible when it is realised that up to one-third of all patients do not take the prescriptions they receive.

Meanwhile, pacemakers in Britain are in shorter supply than dialysis machines. Children are denied critical care because of a shortage of intensive care units in which to treat them. Fifty people die in Merseyside each year for lack of open heart surgery. Many haemophilic children are denied treatment with Factor VIII, which prevents pain from haemorrhage into their joints. And, for some conditions (such as spina bifida), children are simply allowed to die because the cost of treatment is judged to be too high.

In the USA there are no government subsidies for prescriptions except for the very poor. Yet more heart transplants are performed every nine months at Stanford University medical centre in California than have been performed in Britain in the last decade. In 1976 there were more CAT scanners in Houston, Texas (population: about one million) than in all Britain (population 56 million). Yet Britain pioneered scanner technology. Moreover, recent improvements are largely due to the general public, not to the NHS decision-makers. Of the twenty full-body scanners in use in 1979, half were donated to the NHS by individuals and private charitable organisations.

Budget alternatives

To put the magnitude of the contrasts into some perspective, I have made some broad calculations to show what kinds of budget choices are being made by the NHS. Suppose the NHS decided to end its free taxi service and so cut its ambulance budget, say, by 93 per cent. What could be done with these resources?

The NHS could begin by providing dialysis or kidney transplants for every eligible patient (£5000 per patient). It could furnish every major hospital in the country with a CAT scanner, and achieve the same number of scanners *per capita* (about 250 total) as in the USA. This move, incidentally, would save hundreds, perhaps thousands, of additional lives. The NHS would still have enough money left to double the amount spent on the emergency ambulances – to provide them with more equipment and better-trained personnel.

These results could also be achieved by deciding to discontinue "free" GP house calls, "free" eyesight tests and perhaps half of the "free" visits by home nurses and health visitors. They could also be achieved by requiring patients to pay a larger proportion of the cost of the drugs, dentures and eyeglasses they require. Yet decisions such as these are not even seriously considered within the NHS.

A proposed explanation

What accounts for the radical difference in American and British priorities in health care? A possible explanation is that the basic values and preferences of the British and American people are very different. The evidence does not support this conclusion.

The American health care system has been largely shaped by private citizens making choices as individuals in what is, for the most part, a free *market* for health care. In Britain, health care discussions are made through *political* process. If British patients also made individual choices in the private health care system, I believe that British and American priorities would be very similar.

Consider the evidence from those few areas of British health care where patients face money prices – prescriptions, spectacles, and dentures. With predictable consistency, the demand for these items has dropped substantially every time the NHS has raised the fees charged. In 1977 the price charged patients for dentures jumped from £12 to £20. Although £20 is considerably less than the amount paid to dentists (£37), the demand for dentures fell by 29 per cent following the price rise. The evidence suggests that if British patients were paying the full cost, far fewer resources would be devoted to items such as these and more could be channelled to technology such as renal dialysis.

Similar responses by patients would be observed if prices were charged for other NHS services. If patients were required to pay the full cost of GP house calls, I predict that the service would be as rare as it is in the USA. It is, after all, very *wasteful*. The doctor's time is (generally) more valuable than that of his patients. If patients travel to the doctor, they minimise the cost of travel time and allow the doctor to treat more patients. If there is anything seriously wrong with the patient, he goes to the emergency room where the necessary equipment is available to treat him. Few non-acute patients would choose an ambulance over a taxi if they had to pay the full cost of the ambulance ride.

The NHS spends far more on "caring" services than I believe the British public would ever pay out of their own pockets. This does not mean that if British medical care were essentially private, patients would spend less of their income on medical care. They might spend more, as the decreasing spending on "caring" services would be offset by increased spending on "curing" services.

The booming private health care market in Britain is testimony to a steadily growing demand for "curing" services that the NHS either does not offer, or offers at an unacceptably slow place. Private health insurance now covers 2.5 million people; and with the EETPU contract negotiated in 1979, private health insurance has now become a feature of collective bargaining.

Private insurance would spread in Britain

NHS defenders often belittle the significance of the private market for health care by showing that private health insurance covers less than 5 per cent of the population. The number of people covered is remarkable considering that the British public is generally uninformed about the value of such policies. In the USA the high level of patient awareness about medical care is mainly due to the activities of doctors. The doctors themselves inform patients about the value of preventive medicine, the value of CAT scans, the dangers of waiting too long before surgery, etc. In Britain, no comparable activity is taking place, or to the same degree. Who in the NHS has an incentive to tell patients things that will only diminish the stature of the NHS? Even the private insurance companies are enormously restrained in their advertising techniques. In the promotional literature of BUPA you find no mention of NHS patients dying for lack of open-heart surgery or of the dangers of inordinately long waits for NHS surgery. Indeed, BUPA promotional literature contains no criticism of the NHS whatsoever.

Insurance in the USA

Most British citizens also have a highly misleading impression about how the market for private health care works in the USA. The barrage of propaganda coming from the press evokes an image of patients in critical condition being routinely turned away from private hospital emergency rooms because they cannot produce immediate cash or health insurance cards. In the USA, Britons are regularly told, 25 per cent of all personal bankruptcies are due to sickness.

The truth is that it is illegal for a hospital in the USA to deny emergency treatment care to an individual because of inability to pay for treatment. There are, of course, occasional abuses. They make the newspaper headlines precisely because they are so *rare*. They are a small price to pay for avoiding the kind of emergency care received commonly by the *average* NHS patient. British doctors arrive to treat coronary cases an average of four hours after the symptoms begin. By that time, 50 per cent of the patients are dead. (That figure, to give only one source, is from Professor Michael Cooper, *Rationing Health Care*, 1975.)

The number of personal bankruptcies due to sickness in the USA each year is equal to one-twentieth of one per cent of all American families. Many of them are caused because the earning capacity of the patient is impaired rather than because of the medical bills. Moreover, many of the most expensive operations in the USA are performed rarely or not at all in the NHS.

In summary, I believe that the British health care priorities, far from reflecting the true priorities of the British public, reflect the distortions of the political process, which obscure basic values and leads to a very different outcome from the economic market place where choices are made by individual citizens.

Daryl Dixon

Policy Co-ordinator at the Social Welfare Policy Secretariat, a Department of the Commonwealth Government of Australia, in Canberra.

And now a former British Dominion. Australia's standard of living is higher than ours, lower than the American. An Australian public official gives a straightforward account of developments in the financing of Australian health services. For a short period under a Labour Government there was a move towards state insurance. It was soon reversed. The health services are mostly provided by private doctors paid by fees for items of service, in turn based largely on private health insurance, with government subsidies. There is little sign that Australia will copy the NHS and its almost total tax-financing. The outlook is for continuing refinement of financial incentives and payment by patients.

2. AUSTRALIA DOES NOT FOLLOW THE NHS

Recent developments in the financing of Australian health services

This paper reviews developments in the financing of Australian health services over the period 1975 to 1979. It focuses in particular on changes in the distribution of financing between government and private channels and the use of financial incentives to promote cost-consciousness and the effective and efficient allocation of resources.

The paper draws heavily on *A Discussion Paper on Paying for Health Care* by the Australian Hospitals and Health Services Commission (Australian Government Publishing Service, Canberra 1978) and on a subsequent Paper by Dr Sidney Sax (Special Adviser on Social Welfare Policy, Commonwealth of Australia) entitled *Impact of Federal Health Insurance and Health Resource Allocation Policies* in Australia 1975–79, presented to the annual meeting of the American Public Health Association in November 1979.

Firsty it is necessary to describe briefly the organisational and financial context in which these developments have taken place.

The organisational and financial framework for Australian health services

Health expenditure currently accounts for around 8 per cent of Australia's Gross Domestic Product. Most medical care in Australia is provided by private practitioners in return for fees for items of service. The Commonwealth Government has traditionally subsidised the cost of private practitioner services, and most Australians usually avail themselves of private medical insurance to meet a large part of the remaining costs. It has been estimated that in March 1979 around 70 per cent of the Australian population was covered by some form of private health insurance; the proportion has varied over time with changes in the amount and method of supply of government subsidies.

Private practitioners set their own charges, but government subsidies and private health insurance rebates are based on a schedule of fees determined by the Commonwealth Government and periodically reviewed.

State and Territory Governments administer public hospitals, mental health services, public health regulation, licensing and professional registration.

Public hospitals are generally controlled by boards of directors subject to conditions of subsidy determined by the State/Territory health authorities. Their charges for private (usually insured) patients are fixed by the Governments, are uniform throughout Australia and heavily subsidised. Public hospital deficits are shared equally by the Federal and State/Territory governments. Private practitioners treating private patients in public hospitals are paid fees. Anybody who is not a private (insured) patient has a right to treatment in a public hospital as a public patient free of charge, but is cared for by doctors engaged by the hospital.

In private hospitals all patients are treated by their own doctors for fees for items of service. Their hospital charges are determined by the hospital proprietors. The Commonwealth Government subsidises private hospital charges, now at a rate of $16 (about £8) per day.

The Commonwealth Government's heavily subsidised pharmaceutical benefits scheme makes listed pharmaceutical items available free of charge to pensioners and at a charge of $2.75 (about £1.40) per item for other patients.

Another important Commonwealth Government subsidy scheme covers medical care in nursing homes.

The cost of most community based ancillary health care services are shared dollar-for-dollar by the Commonwealth and State/Territory Governments.

Recent developments in financing Australian health services

The financing of Australian health services has been changed since 1975 as governments, and their priorities, have changed. Governments seeking to ensure the provision of health services of high quality and ready accessibility for their citizens have had to come to terms with harsh economic and budgetary difficulties.

Government involvement in the financing of health services reached its zenith with the (Labour) Commonwealth Government's 1975 Medibank Scheme which aimed at more universal provision of health services and provided for:

(i) 85 per cent of the scheduled fee for any item of medical service to be covered by tax-financed benefits, subject to a maximum patient co-payment of $5.00 per item, with no contribution generally being required from aged pensioners or the poor; and

(ii) free inpatient and outpatient medical care in public hospitals for patients who chose public care, regardless of their means.

Mainly as a result of this scheme, the proportion of health expenditures borne by the government sector rose from 62 per cent in 1974–75 to 72 per cent in 1975–76. Private sector spending fell from 38 per cent of the total to 28 per cent. Total (private and public) health expenditures grew by 35 per cent in 1975–76 following a 39.9 per cent increase in 1974–75.

The Liberal Commonwealth Government which took office in December 1975 espoused a policy of rigorous restraint in government expenditures as a means of reducing the extremely high rates of inflation (about 16 per cent a year).

Significant success in expenditure control was made possible by alterations in 1976 to the agreements with the States/Territories for the sharing of public hospital operating costs. Instead of paying half of the audited net costs whatever these turned out to be, the Commonwealth Government assumed the right to approve budgets in advance, to question over-expenditures or shortfalls in anticipated revenue collections, and finally to pay half of only "approved" net operating costs. In effect, cost-"caps" were applied. Because financial tax resources are limited at their source, health authorities have had little alternative but to impose increasing tight systems of control over public operating costs.

The result was that the annual growth in real terms of public hospital operating costs declined from 11.2 per cent in 1975–76 to 8.8 per cent in 1976–77, 6.2 per cent in 1977–78 and 3.4 per cent in 1978–79. Zero real growth in operating costs is the target for 1979–80.

The history of the Commonwealth Government's medical benefits arrangements since 1975 has been complex. Change has followed change in quick succession:

In October 1976 the:

(i) abolition of universal tax-financed benefits paid by a single Commonwealth agency; and

(ii) introduction of a health insurance levy on taxable income with fixed annual ceilings on an individual's contribution and exemptions for the poor and people who purchased combined medical/hospital cover from private health insurance funds. (The funds became subject to firm regulation by the Commonwealth Department and could not reject subscribers. People without private insurance retained their right to free medical care at public hospitals).

In July 1978 the reduction of basic medical benefits from 85 per cent to 75 per cent and the increase in the maximum patient co-payment from $5 to $10.

In November 1978:

(i)   the abolition of the health insurance levy;

(ii)   introduction of a new universal government medical benefit of 40 per cent of the scheduled medical fee for any item of medical service, subject to a maximum patient co-payment of $20 (medical care at public hospitals remained free of charge for people without private insurance who chose treatment by doctors engaged by the hospital);

(iii) provision of additional voluntary health insurance cover by the private funds;

(iv)   full settlement by the Commonwealth Government of private medical bills of most aged pensioners and the "disadvantaged" at the reduced rate of 85 per cent and 75 per cent of the scheduled fees respectively.

In September 1979, government benefit on schedule fees of less than $20 for any item of medical service was abolished but the Commonwealth Government undertook payment of the full amount in excess of $20 up to the limit of the schedule fee. No changes were made to public hospital arrangements or to the system of paying for private medical services for pensioners and the disadvantaged. (It is estimated that in March 1979 10 per cent of the Australian population were covered by the arrangements for pensioners. Reliable figures are not yet available on the numbers covered by the arrangements for the "disadvantaged".)

Voluntary additional private health insurance cover has become even more important. The private funds (with Commonwealth Government encouragement) have greatly widened the range of available insurance cover by offering varying levels of co-insurance and co-payment, and one fund has created a number of schemes incorporating deductibles (no contribution by the fund until bills in a year exceed specified amounts).

The impact of changes in financing arrangements

The rapid pace of change in Australian health financing in recent years has made it difficult to collect comparable data or evaluate the effects of the changes. What can be said from the latest available aggregate figures is that there has been:

(i) a decline in the rate of growth of total health expenditure (from 39.9 per cent in 1974–75 to an estimated 10.7 per cent in 1977–78);

(ii) a reduction in the share of total health expenditures borne by government (from 72 per cent in 1975–76 to 62 per cent in 1977–78);

(iii) a compensating increase in the share borne by individuals (from 28 per cent in 1975–76 to 38 per cent in 1977–78).

Precise analysis of the reasons for the decline in total health expenditure growth is not possible but the following factors have contributed:

(i) reductions in the rate of wage and price inflation;

136

(ii) the cost-"caps" applied to public hospital operating costs;
(iii) growth and price controls on nursing homes;
and (more speculatively):
(iv) reduced government subsidies for private medical care.

Prospects

Time will tell whether the September 1979 arrangements prove sustainable. A number of concerns have been expressed:

(i) that recent increases in private health insurance rates will prompt many healthy persons to opt not to insure, thus (by leaving health insurance funds with a higher proportion of high-cost chronically-ill contributors) setting off further rounds of rate increases and threatening the financial viability of health insurance funds;

(ii) that these developments will be exacerbated because some people, not understanding the complexities of the choices to be made, will not insure;

(iii) that the financial position of many general practitioners will be eroded by increases in the number of uninsured people who seek treatment as socially disadvantaged persons (and have their bills met by the Commonwealth Government at the reduced rate of 75 per cent of the schedule fee) or as public hospital outpatients;

(iv) that, with current high levels of medical manpower, general practitioners will bolster their financial position by over-servicing insured patients;

(v) that many persons will do without necessary medical services thus risking theirs and their families' future health;

(vi) that high-income earners will take a "free-ride" by not insuring and relying on Commonwealth medical benefits and free care in public hospitals.

Despite these concerns, careful monitoring of developments rather than precipitate change seems called for in the immediate future. It is hoped that a recently-established Commission of Inquiry into the Efficiency and Administration of Hospitals will provide more acceptable answers to some of the seemingly intractable problems of Australian health service financing. But it seems likely that a combination of administrative controls and financial incentives will continue to be applied.

Arthur Seldon

Finally, a European country, with, in the North, Western culture and, in the South, a agrarian society, and a lower average living standard than in the Britain, although the gap is narrowing. In January 1980 Italy introduced what it calls "a National Health Service". So far it exists only on paper, and that is where it will largely remain. It will not follow the structure of the British National Health Service. Essay XXIII, based on a Paper delivered at a recent conference in Rome, argues that the British experience shows why Italy will not develop the "National Health Service" it has devised, and why it would be unwise to make the attempt.

3. ITALY: WARNED IN TIME?

Introduction

Ever since the British National Health Service was created in 1948, its advocates have claimed it was "the envy of the world". Yet no country has copied it – until 1 January 1980. None outside the communist world had full state control of the organisation and financing of medical care.

Since 1 January 1980, Italy has been the only Western country to copy the British NHS. The main features – on paper – are the same. The differences are secondary. Both systems are financed by taxation. Everything else flows from that. And if this main feature is not soon changed in Italy, the same consequences will follow in Italy as we in Britain have witnessed in our country.

Italy and Britain

The two countries have differences in culture, economic structure and history. And supporters of the Italian "National Health Service" *hope* it will work differently from the NHS. The supporters of the new system also point to new techniques developed by American and British economists to monitor the working and effectiveness of the Italian "National Health Service" by "health indicators".

All this is possible. But the voices that Italy should heed are those that emphasise realism rather than optimistic conjecture. For this realism is based on experience in Britain: the British NHS is a warning to Italy. The optimistic conjectures are based on theoretical hypothesis which are untested by experience or experimentation.

Against the optimistic conjectures, I emphasise the realistic view that the consequences of the National Health Service in Britain would be expected to appear in Italy. If the optimistic conjectures are allowed to dominate thinking in Italy the undesirable consequences will be *more* likely to appear than if the Italian politicians and bureaucrats are aware of the effects of the British National Health Service in the thirty years since 1948.

Market failure is curable; government failure is incurable

As with the British NHS, the Italian "National Health Service" has supporters among intellectuals – economists and others – whose case for *state* medicine rest largely on the case against *private* medicine in the market. The intellectual case against private medicine in 1980 is more than it was in Britain in 1948. There are four main arguments of "market failure".

First, the "agency relationship"; the doctor is the expert whom the patient as amateur has to use as his "agent" to advise on treatment. The doctor is then empowered to advise on more treatment, or more expensive treatment, than the patient "needs".

Secondly, in private medicine in the market where private insurance reimburses the patient he is induced to use more costly treatment than he really "needs" because he is not paying for each item as it occurs.

Thirdly, "externalities"; medical care may indirectly affect third parties external to the two directly involved – the doctor and patient. It may confer benefits (such as reduced exposure to infection) which are ignored by the two parties.

Fourthly, "monopoly"; doctors can restrict entry to new students by laying down unnecessarily high standards or exerting pressure on governments.

All these four causes of market failure may make the supply of market care different from the optimum. But by themselves they do not make a decisive case for a national health service.

The economics of politics

I base my views about the *likely* consequences of the Italian NHS on the judgement that more important than these technical/economic weaknesses of "market failure" are the economics of public finance and politics of which Italian economists were prominent among the early pioneers – Vilfredo Pareto, Gaetano Mosca, Antonio De Viti De Marco, Amilcare Puviani and Mauro Fasiani.

This approach produces a *realistic* as opposed to a conjectural analysis of what is likely to happen when medicine passes into the ultimate control of politicians and bureaucrats because its financing is derived from central taxation. Before I say what is *likely* to happen in the Italian National Health Service, I would reject the argument of its supporters on three grounds:

(i) The technical/economic analysis of "market failure" is not as strong as its exponents seem to think. Even if the causes of "market failure" were unavoidable, the effects tend to cancel out. The "agency relationship" and "moral hazard" tend to enlarge the output of medical care. Externalities and monopoly tend to restrict it.

(ii) None of the four sources of market failure is inevitable. "Moral hazard" can be controlled by enabling patients to pay a part of the cost of each item of treatment. These methods vary from the re-imbursement systems well known in Europe – France, Sweden etc. to deductibles (in which the patient pays the first part of each bill) or co-insurances (in which the patient pays a proportion of each bill) common in the U.S.A. "Moral" hazard is worst of all in the NHS where there is no payment at all.

The "agency relationship" – the power of the doctor to mislead the patient – is unavoidably effective only *in extremis* where there is no time to question the doctor's emergency advice or treatment. In other conditions, the patient is not at the mercy of the doctor because he can take a "second opinion". The patient's safeguard against a doctor is the existence of all other doctors. Family doctors also tend to become medical "brokers" who advise on the best specialist. And information about good and bad doctors spreads quickly.

"Externalities" can also be "internalised" by subsidising medical treatments, such as early attention to infection disease.

Monopoly among doctors can be disciplined by removing their power to restrict entry. This is most difficult in state medicine.

(iii) These problems are made even *worse* when all medical care is put into the control of government. Government, in practice, means politicians (which means party politics) and bureaucrats (whose interests may conflict with the interests of patients).

Yet these political influences have had very little discussion in Italy recently (and too little in Britain). It is easy to see why. All forms of medical care that evolve spontaneously seem slow to the academic, who is often by nature a "social engineer". He has the best of intentions to improve the lot of his fellow men by large-scale organisation that appears to offer the prospect of raising health standards more quickly, with less duplication of services, prompt attention to people with low incomes or regions with agrarian industry. In the midst of this euphoria, the realities are apt to be forgotten, ignored or minimised.

A realistic view of the consequences

Both in Britain and Italy the supporters of the National Health Service in each country make very large but unsupported claims. There is a wide gap between claims and performance – between textbook theory and day-to-day real life. The theory says the Italian "National Health Service" will (at some time in the future):
  (i) replace two hundred or so insurance funds with one national source of finance – earmarked taxation to cover everyone;
 (ii) supply all medical care – except "inessential" drugs – equally and "free";
(iii) administer the system by regional authorities;
(iv) distribute medical resources more equitably between the regions, especially between the industrial North and the Mezzogiorno;
 (v) control costs to avoid excessive services and give better value for money.
   I reply that commonsense, the logic of political institutions, and the British experience indicate that the Italian "National Health Service" will achieve *none* of these objectives.

1. It will *not* cover everyone by medical care financed by earmarked taxation.
   (a) As incomes rise, more Italians will seek in the market better medical care than the state can supply equally for all.
   (b) The increased taxation will be increasingly avoided or evaded because no Italian will receive better care for his family by paying higher taxes (or receive less medical care for his family by paying less taxes).
   (c) The taxation "earmarked" for the National Health Service will either be a lower percentage of the Gross Domestic Product than Italian citizens would *voluntarily* have spent, or it will be "raided" when other national requirements are regarded by the government as even more urgent – such as strengthening the national defences if the death of Tito had invited Russian invasion.
   (d) Although for the first time the *total* (national) cost of medical care will be known, the information on the cost of *each* medical treatment will be destroyed, so that the allocation of resources will be arbitrary.
   (e) Firms will find they cannot afford to lose their men who have to fit into "the system" and will make arrangements to cover them by private insurance for private medical attention.
2. The Italian National Health Service will *not* supply medical care "free". It will exact increasing taxes for deteriorating services. By *appearing* to supply medical care "free', it will destroy the bargaining power of the patient (and thus expose him to the worst form of agency relationship), make the doctor increasingly dependent on the state for his income, and worsen the personal voluntary relationship between doctor and patient, who will lose respect for each other because they will find it more difficult to escape from each other.
   Neither will the Italian "National Health Service" supply medical care equally. It will supply it in accordance with personal influence or group pressure based on cultural, social, occupational, economic or political power. The poor, the inarticu-

late, the incapacitated (especially the old and the mentally ill, as in Britain) and the weak will receive less than the better off, the articulate, the capable and the bully.

3. The Italian National Health Service will *not* in practice be administered by *regional* "authorities" with effective autonomous power to supply medical care to suit their regions, but by regional executors of *central* government policy. As long as the *finance* is raised by central government, the regions will have their *orders* from the central government.

4. The Italian National Health Service will *not* redistribute resources more equitably from regions of less "medical need" to regions of more "medical need" for the same reason as in 3 above, and additionally because the politicians in power will use the tax funds to favour medical services in regions where they can reap *electoral* advantage (*as in Britain*).

5. The Italian "National Health Service" will *not* control costs by bringing them down to the optimal amount for services the people want. It will use its buying power with doctors, nurses, administrators, manual workers, pharmaceutical firms, appliance, building and other suppliers to "squeeze" them and bring costs down *too far*. The reason is that cutting costs will be to the *short*-term electoral advantage of politicians in power, and they will not be concerned about the *long*-term effects on the quality of staff, equipment or buildings. But the patient will be harmed by deterioration in the quality.

The Italian Minister of Health has been given an impossible task. For all these reasons he will *not* be able to provide the services required to satisfy the grandiose expectations aroused by the publicity – now on the walls of Italian cities. Italians will before long become dissatisfied, disillusioned, and cynical not only about their "National Health Service" but also about Italian politicians and Italian democracy.

XXII
Why the NHS Must Fail

Arthur Seldon

The concluding essay argues that the NHS will suffer increasing strain as rising incomes enable more and more people to pay for better – because more personal – medical care than the state can provide out of taxation. The NHS will therefore be able to keep itself going only by more coercion of doctors and nurses to work in it, of patients to accept it, and of taxpayers to continue paying for it. But doctors and nurses will want to maintain high professional standards, patients will want better service, taxpayers will see no reason to pay for deteriorating service. If private – and therefore better – medicine is repressed, doctors will increasingly emigrate, patients will seek treatment overseas, taxpayers will avoid or evade taxes. The British people will not accept second-rate medical service except by coercion. And they will not accept coercion.

Introduction

The NHS must fail to supply the British people with the best medical care they want because it prevents them as individual consumers from paying for the services that suit their personal family requirements, circumstances and preferences.

This judgement is common sense. It reflects a first principle of economics that people will pay more for higher quality. And it is the lesson of political experience.

Common sense, economics and politics

The NHS has flouted, and continues to flout, all three: common sense, economics, and political experience. It must continue to flout them because it is based on a principle that denies all three. Common sense, economics and politics teach that individuals will sacrifice more of other satisfactions, will pay more for a service that benefits them, their families, or others they love, than for a service that is indifferent to their wishes or even feelings. And this means they will pay more if they can pay by a method that produces better services than by a method that does not. This fundamental weakness was acknowledged by two Labour ministers after experience of financing social services: Douglas (now Lord) Houghton and the late R. H. S. Crossman.

The NHS forces people to pay by a method – taxation – that cuts the connection between amount paid and quality of service. No man in Britain can do anything for himself, or his wife, or children, or parents, or friends (or strangers) he wants to help in sickness by paying more taxes.

The way in which he could ensure better attention is by paying for each item of service, or to each doctor, or clinic, or hospital, for a period. The wealthy can pay out-of-pocket. For most people individual payment of this kind can be arranged by insurance.

The NHS dilemma: the divorce of payment from service

But the NHS is caught in a dilemma from which there is no escape. It is based on the very principle of *divorcing* payment from service. This, its supporters say, is its glory: that no-one has to pay anything at all (with minor exceptions) at the time of service. But this method of payment, or non-payment, we can now see, is also its fatal weakness. The NHS is caught in a tragic dilemma. It cannot, by taxation, raise enough money to provide people with the health services they would like, and would pay for; yet it prevents people paying more to obtain better services.

That is why the NHS must fail, no matter how much longer it is held together by exhortation and coercion. It ceaselessly appeals to the dedication of doctors and nurses, to the trade union solidarity of employees concerned about their jobs as the quality of their service continues to fall, and to the political sympathy of ordinary people with the original noble objective of a service in which no-one, especially the poor, would have to think about the grubby necessity of money when ill.

The NHS will fail because all three cements are dissolving. The dedication of doctors and nurses is under increasing strain as the older generation is replaced by younger people increasingly paid by the state as public officials rather than by patients as providers of a personal service. The solidarity of trade union employees will be under increasing strain as the public resists rising taxes for deteriorating quality. And the public sympathy for a noble service is wearing thin as it clashes with the concern of individuals for their families in sickness.

Rejection of the NHS

Most of all, the NHS will fail because its method of financing cannot provide medical services that keep pace with the desire and ability of more and more British people for better quality that the state can supply equally (or rather try to supply equally, for it fails) out of taxation. More and more ordinary people will be able to express their elemental instinctive urge to ensure the comfort of a child in pain, reassure a wife anxious about a symptom, or save a parent neglected in a large ward. And they will put these intensely personal anxieties before the political appeal to continue supporting a system that *prevents them acting as human beings* – as parents, husbands or children.

The dilemma of the NHS is that, if it tried to satisfy these human anxieties by giving better service (which means prompter, more sensitive, more personal, more convenient in time or place, more comfortable, etc.) to people who transferred funds from other expenditures by paying more, it would be destroying the very principle that was supposed to make it better than all other medical systems in the first place. A NHS that, to save itself from deterioration, encouraged people to pay more for better service would have to offer *varying* qualities. It would then no longer be – or aim to be – a *uniform*, equal service for all whatever they paid. In an effort to maintain its very existence, it would have destroyed itself. From that dilemma there is no escape except increasing coercion of doctors and nurses to continue providing deteriorating service, increasing coercion of patients to accept it, and increasing coercion of taxpayers to pay for it. The NHS confronts intensifying coercion or eventual collapse.

The two causes of inequality

Not only double but multiple standards are the only way to raise standards for all – *especially the poorest*. The search for an equal-service NHS is vain as long as people differ, as long as they put their loved ones before abstract political dogmas, as long as incomes differ, and as long as incomes rise. The whole issue of equality has been confused with that of poverty; and both have obscured the overriding objective of liberty.

Inequality in access to medical care arises from two causes. The first, emphasised by the obsessive egalitarians, is that of inequality of incomes, "poverty", inability to pay. But that is an obstacle that can be increasingly surmounted, by methods constantly explored in Britain and other countries from the British Family Income Supplement, through the Australian topping-up of low incomes (to enable the poor to have a choice of health insurance and doctor or hospital), to the American idea of the voucher recommended to the Department of Health most recently by the Ambassador in Britain.

The second cause of unequal access to medicine, ignored by the egalitarians, is the *readiness* to pay more for better medicine. Many in Britain would pay more, but the NHS stops them. Yet this is the great hope for the future: that more and more people will *voluntarily* spend more than the state now allows them to do. And that will be the source of the additional funds for medicine. The method of the NHS is compulsion – taxation. The hope for British medicine, and for British health, is that British doctors, nurses and administrators can make themselves so good, as they have been in the past, that the British people will want to pay them more voluntarily.

The NHS has vainly strained for equality, and thereby denied medicine the funds that would have improved it for all. The egalitarian philosophy has never understood that, where there are no winners, all – *especially the poor* – are losers.

It can be only a matter of years before the NHS strait-jacket succumbs to social and economic change, whatever the politicians in power want, or think. So far they have hoped to save it by re-organisation: decentralising this function, centralising that one; adding a layer here, lopping off a layer there; strengthening expertise (as the professionals want) by increasing the power or authority of appointed experts on local or regional bodies, or strengthening democracy (as the politicians want) by increasing the power or authority of elected representatives (Councillors or others). The 1980 reforms will fail likewise.

All to no avail. All this re-organisation of administration or management is guessing in the dark and ignoring the real engine of improvement: *the flow of money*. Improvement will come only by motivating *individuals* – doctors, nurses, administrators, etc. – by varying the resources at their disposal according to the effectiveness with which they use them. This means channelling funds for equipment and buildings to the individuals who make the most of them for the good of the patient. But it also includes additional payment – fees, salaries, wages, allowances – to *individual* doctors, nurses and administrators for good work and diminished payment for bad work.

A beautiful carriage – but where's the ruddy horse?

The NHS has lived on its noble aims for too long. It was designed as a beautiful carriage, based on compassion, dedication, public service. All these motives can be expressed as much as individuals are capable. And they appear most strongly in times of crisis and emergency, when preventing pain and saving life is the supreme aim and everything else is, for the time, secondary.

One day selfless dedication may suffice for medicine, and do the rest of the world's work. Until that day, there are only two other methods: state coercion or individual inducement. Coercion is required for "public health" – the "public" goods of environmental and preventive services that people in a free society voluntarily agree through their democratic institutions to pay "compulsorily" by taxation because they cannot be refused to people who refuse to pay – "free riders" would not bear their share of the cost. Here is where the NHS mistake was made. If it had confined itself to *public* health (and left a different government department to deal with income and poverty), it might have succeeded. But it set out to embrace *all* health services. That is where it went wrong.

Not all health services are public goods. Many or most hospital services, most family doctor services, drugs and appliances are essentially personal services for which people can (and would wish to) pay more for better quality. This is the large part of medical care that requires encouragement (by better payment) for individuals to do their best – and discouragement, by patients moving elsewhere, for individuals who do not do their best. This, therefore, is the large scope for paying for medicine by fees for doctors and others, charges for services, prices for medicines, etc. backed by insurance.

The NHS is, or was, a beautiful carriage that is not getting very far because it lacks the horsepower of individual incentive to the supplier to serve the customer. To adapt

146

Roy Campbell's lines in 1930 to 1980 NHS loyalists:
You use the snaffle and the curb alright,
But where's the bloody horse?

Four problems to tackle

There will be problems to solve. We shall have to do what is possible to deal with four possible causes of "market failure". Monopoly and "social benefits" (to third parties) tend to restrict the production of medical care below the optimum. "Moral hazard" (that people will demand more if insurance pays the bill) and the "agency relationship" (which may tempt the doctor as expert "agent" to advise unnecessary treatment to the amateur patient) tend to expand production above the optimum. The only effective solutions are the maximum possible competition between suppliers by more effective anti-monopoly law, and the maximum possible information, not least by announcements and advertising as the American Medical Association is beginning to welcome so that consumers can "shop" and choose between doctors and hospitals. (Discussed more fully in Essay XXI.)

These solutions are imperfect, but all four problems are even more severe and more difficult to remove where medicine is under state control The state is a monopoly far exceeding all private (and therefore limited) monopolies, whether of doctors, nurses, trade unions, or pharmaceutical firms. The social benefits of private medicine can be dealt with by financial encouragement to services that do good to people generally; but there is no outside compunction on politicians or bureaucrats to deal with the external effects of the medical services they control. Moral hazard is even worse in the NHS, which cannot charge for services to cover the costs of varying quality. And the "agency relationship" is even more subject to abuse in state-controlled monopoly medicine from which patients cannot escape at all.

All these problems must be faced and tackled. And other Western countries are facing and tackling them. They arise from the human and technical nature of the supply and of the demand for medical care under all systems – state or private. They are not faced or tackled by the NHS, but swept under the carpet. Since 1948 they have been ignored, but they have festered. They must be faced and tackled in the 1980s by radical reform of medical financing.

Conclusion

The path to better medical services for Britain is the radical transformation of the way in which it is financed. The NHS cannot improve, and must fail, because its "free" financing, which destroys information, is its heart, without which it dies. That is why, whatever the difficulties, Britain must now find ways to finance medicine that enable *individual* people to pay for better services. More funds will then be channelled by all the people to medical care as a whole, the quality of British medicine will improve, the people will have the services they want, and the health of the British will benefit.

Government can hold the NHS together only by increasing coercion of doctors and patients. If government does not recognise the British people's ability and readiness to pay for something better, they will find it outside in private medicine at home or overseas. But public opinion could embolden government into removing the coercion and the obstacles to the voluntary evolution of medical care that suits both doctors and patients.